Snoring and Sleep Apnea

Sleep Well, Feel Better

Snoring and Sleep Apnea

Sleep Well, Feel Better

Ralph A. Pascualy, M.D.

Sally Warren Soest, M.S.

Third Edition

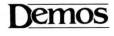

New York

Demos Medical Publishing, Inc., 386 Park Avenue South, New York, New York 10016

Made in Canada.

Illustrations: Robert Holmberg, University of Washington,
Health Sciences Center for Educational Resources

Photographs: 6.1, 6.2, 6.3, 6.4, 6.5, 6.6 by Gayle Rieber Photography
7.1 (A) from video by Dr. Stephen B. Anderson
7.2 Photographs courtesy of:
(A) Mallinckrodt Nellcor Puritan Bennett, Inc.
(B) Respironics, Inc.
(C), (D), and (F) ResMed Corp.
(E) DeVilbiss (Sunrise Medical)
(GE) Fisher & Paykel
7.3 Photographs courtesy of:
(A) Mallinckrodt Nellcor Puritan Bennett, Inc.
(B), (C), (D), and (E) ResMed Corp.
(F) Respironics, Inc.
7.4 OPAP Corporation
7.7 (A, B) courtesy of Dr. Nelson Powell
9.1, 9.2, 14.1 courtesy of ResCare, Ltd. ResMed Corp.

Video capture: 7.1 (A, B) Joseph Wilmhoff, University of Washington,
Health Sciences Center for Educational Resources.

Library of Congress Cataloging-in-Publication Data
Pascualy, Ralph A., 1951–
    Snoring and sleep apnea: sleep well, feel better / Ralph A. Pascualy,
Sally Warren Soest. — 3rd ed.
        p.   cm.
    Prev. ed. had subtitle: Personal and family guide to diagnosis and treatment.
    Includes bibliographical references and index.
    ISBN 1-888799-29-3 (softcover)
    1. Sleep apnea syndromes — Popular works. 2. Snoring — Popular works.
I. Soest, Sally Warren, 1942–   . II. Title.
RC737.5 .P37 2000
616.8′498—dc21   00-031445

Contents

Foreword

Sleep apnea syndrome is number one among the hundred-plus sleep disorders recognized today. Why?

1. Sleep apnea is common: it affects one in ten middle-aged men. It is slightly less common in women.

2. Sleep apnea, untreated, can be deadly.

3. Sleep apnea patients are poorly diagnosed and treated because of the lack of trained sleep experts.

Sleep apnea robs people of vitality, health, and sometimes life itself. Loss of vitality will be familiar to many readers of this book. People suffering from sleep apnea fall asleep anywhere and everywhere, even while driving. Their heavy snoring disrupts their own sleep and often that of their family. They drag themselves to work despite exhaustion, doze at their desks, stumble home completely drained, and fall asleep on the sofa. They lack the energy to enjoy family life or the company of friends.

The health consequences of sleep apnea are even more grave. Untreated sleep apnea puts people at high risk for driving accidents, high blood pressure, stroke, irregular heart rhythms, and other life-threatening complications.

Treatment is available and dramatically effective. Formerly sick, sleepy people quickly regain their vigor, resume their cherished activities, and thrive. Life is restored.

Accurate diagnosis is the major problem. Eighty percent to 90 percent of sleep apnea victims are still undiagnosed. The National Commission on Sleep Disorders Research heard countless witnesses testify to suffering for 10 years or more before sleep apnea was correctly diagnosed and treated.

My primary mission in life today is to lift the shroud of darkness surrounding sleep disorders, and with it years of prolonged and needless suffering. Education is the key—public education, patient education, and medical education.

This book answers all three of those educational needs. It educates the sleep apnea sufferer and the public alike. Further, the book is an authoritative survey of sleep apnea diagnosis and treatment for the primary care physician.

Ralph Pascualy and Sally Soest have produced a much needed guide for people who suspect they have sleep apnea, for people who have been diagnosed, and for those undertaking lifelong treatment.

I can recommend this book to all those with sleep apnea and their friends and families. Use it as a pathfinder. Let it point the way out of the twilight of sleep apnea to timely diagnosis, appropriate treatment, and a bright future.

William C. Dement, M.D., Ph.D.
Chairman, National Commission on Sleep Disorders Research
Palo Alto, California

Preface

The Inspiration

This book was born in the convergence of two separate viewpoints—doctor and patient. One of the authors (SWS) is married to a person who has sleep apnea. The other author (RAP) is the sleep disorders specialist who diagnosed and treated him. The two authors met across an information gap. They wrote this book in a combined effort to bridge that gap.

The need for this book was clear to Sally Soest from the day her husband heard, by chance, about sleep apnea: a newspaper story told of a truck driver who kept falling asleep at the wheel. Seeking additional information, the author discovered that little was written about sleep apnea except in specialized sleep medicine journals. Sleep apnea was surrounded by an information vacuum — scant public awareness, no guideposts for the patient, and poor recognition even in the medical community.

The author learned that this absence of information has a price. A surprising 20 million Americans have this potentially fatal disorder, yet 90 percent are still undiagnosed. Some of those unsuspecting people will die prematurely from the effects of unrecognized, untreated sleep apnea — a high price to pay for lack of information.

As the author met other sleep apnea patients, she became aware of a typical pattern. The most common means of diagnosis seemed to be self-diagnosis by chance, by the patient himself or by a loved one. However, before that many people spent years seeking the correct diagnosis while doctors treated the symptoms — without associating them with sleep apnea. For his heavy snoring, a patient might be advised to try a decongestant or to tell his wife to sleep in the guest room. For his weight problems, he might be told, "Lose weight." For his heart problems, he might receive a prescription for heart medication; for his drowsiness, a stimulant; for his sleep complaints, a sleeping pill. Meanwhile the patient felt worse, and the untreated sleep apnea progressed.

Once a person has received a diagnosis of sleep apnea, the absence of reliable patient support literature has left him without the means to understand this complex disorder, to choose the appropriate treatment, and to deal with long-term issues.

As a sleep disorders specialist, Ralph Pascualy has struggled continually to fill the sleep apnea information vacuum, trying both to provide meaningful patient education material and to raise the level of awareness within the medical community.

The two authors agreed that it was time for a clear, authoritative book written for people with actual or suspected sleep apnea, for their spouses, and for family doctors alike, to help them understand sleep apnea and lead them toward more timely diagnosis and appropriate, successful treatment.

*T*he Message

- Sleep apnea is:
  surprisingly common,
  debilitating,
  potentially fatal,
  treatable, and
  frequently unrecognized by family doctors.
- If you have the symptoms described in Chapter 1, act now. Take the initiative, schedule a sleep test, and find out if you have sleep apnea.
- Don't waste your prime years. Treatment of sleep apnea can restore health and vigor so you have the energy to do the things you enjoy in life.
- Have your sleep test done by a qualified sleep specialist.

*W*hat This Book Will Do for You

As our system of medical care evolves, medical costs increase, managed care becomes more prevalent, and patients face new challenges to obtain the care they need. Patients need to be well-informed consumers and ready to be assertive about receiving the appropriate diagnostic tests and the most effective treatments. The information in this book will arm you to be an effective sleep apnea consumer.

The following chapters describe the causes and consequences of sleep apnea, the tests for diagnosing sleep apnea, and pros and cons of current treatments.

Chapter 12 tells how to find a qualified sleep specialist and the nearest accredited sleep testing center.

Chapters 13 through 15 contain suggestions about living with sleep apnea and dealing with the treatment process, plus information on products and services for people who are being treated for sleep apnea.

The names of patients have been changed to preserve their privacy. In the interest of simplicity and because sleep apnea is more common among males, patients usually have been referred to as "he" and their partners as "she." This should not be interpreted to imply any disregard for the many women who have sleep apnea and their caring, supportive male partners.

You can free yourself from the twilight world of lifeless days and tortured nights. Make an appointment at the nearest accredited sleep center. Do it now!

Ralph A. Pascualy, M.D.
Sally Warren Soest, M.S.
Seattle, Washington

chapter 1

Do You Have Sleep Apnea?

What Is Sleep Apnea?

Sleep apnea (pronounced "AP-nee-uh") is a breathing disorder that affects people while they sleep, usually without their knowing it. The most common symptom is loud, heavy snoring, which is often treated as a joke. But sleep apnea is no joking matter, for it can often result in heart problems, automobile accidents, strokes, and death. Sleep apnea is a potentially fatal disorder.

People with sleep apnea stop breathing repeatedly during a night's sleep. [The word *apnea* comes from the Greek prefix *a* ("no") and the Greek word *pnoia* ("breath").] Breathing may stop 10, 20, or even 100 or more times per hour of sleep and may not start again for a minute or longer. As you can imagine, these sleep/breathing disruptions deprive the person of both sleep and oxygen.

This may not sound terribly serious. "So what?" you may think. "So the person is a little tired or sleepy during the day. What's the problem?"

The problem is twofold. First, sleep apnea is a serious health hazard. Second, a stunning number of people have sleep apnea and don't know it — between 20 million and 25 million Americans. In a recent study of 30- to 60-year-olds, 24 percent of the men and 9 percent of the women had signs of sleep apnea.[1]

A disturbing study of a group of truckers showed that 87 percent had signs of sleep apnea.[2] This is a tragedy in the making because people with untreated sleep apnea are at high risk of falling asleep at the wheel, and when a trucker dies behind the wheel, he sends an average of 4.3 innocent victims to their graves.

Unless it is properly treated, sleep apnea can cause:

- Irregular heartbeat
- High blood pressure
- Enlargement of the heart
- Increased risk of heart failure
- Increased risk of stroke
- Excessive sleepiness
- Workplace and automobile accidents
- Impotence
- Uncontrollable weight gain
- Psychological symptoms, such as irritability and depression
- Deterioration of memory, alertness, and coordination
- Death

Untreated sleep apnea can be progressive, worsening over the course of 10 or 20 years, until it presents a real threat to life.

C A S E   S T U D Y

On the Wednesday before Christmas 1985, Reverend Allen felt himself slipping toward death. This 67-year-old retired minister had seen one doctor after another, searching for the reason for his declining health. Specialists had treated him for heart problems and a variety of other symptoms. But no one had been able to explain what was causing his problems. By December 1985, Mr. Allen was so weak he could hardly walk across his living room.

Now his only prayer was that he might make it through Christmas.

Mr. Allen had lacked energy all his life; even a little exertion wore him out. He slept poorly and never awakened refreshed. When he retired from preaching, he had looked forward to getting plenty of rest and finally feeling better. Instead he had felt more exhausted than ever. His health had become much worse.

He began to lose his coordination. Simple things, such as walking and writing, became difficult. His memory was failing and he would forget familiar words. This embarrassed and saddened him, for he had been a skilled craftsman with words, a preacher's most powerful tools. But now those tools seemed scattered and lost. Even his sense of humor had disappeared. The previous summer his wife had noticed a story in an insurance company magazine about a disorder called sleep apnea. The symptoms had rung a familiar bell — heavy snoring, daytime sleepiness, and exhaustion. She had awakened Mr. Allen, who was asleep as usual in his easy chair, and suggested that he might find the article interesting.

Indeed he did! The article described him exactly. Excited and hopeful, Mr. Allen took the article to his doctor. But his doctor was not particularly interested.

The next six months became a race with time as Mr. Allen's health rapidly deteriorated. His wife doggedly pursued their only lead — sleep apnea — through a long string of discouraging phone calls. Finally, they were put in touch with a new sleep disorders center in a nearby city. They made an appointment for an interview on the Wednesday before Christmas.

On the appointment day Mr. Allen seemed so frail that his wife was afraid he might die on the way to the sleep center. She nearly canceled the appointment. But Mr. Allen was determined to try to make it through Christmas. "What's the difference," he had shrugged, "whether you go to Heaven from home or from the freeway?"

The sleep specialist immediately suspected severe sleep apnea. He rearranged his schedule so that Mr. Allen could have a sleep test the very next night. The doctor knew that if he delayed, he would be sorry for a very long time.

Sleep tests revealed that Mr. Allen had severe obstructive sleep apnea. He was immediately started on treatment with CPAP, a breathing device that is used during sleep (see Chapter 7).

"And that," says Mr. Allen, "was a new beginning! The first morning after I went on CPAP, I woke up feeling refreshed. I wanted to take a walk!"

Three months later, this man who had been near death, barely able to shuffle across his living room, was walking three-quarters of a mile every day. And, to his friends' delight and his own, his sense of humor had returned.

Reverend Allen's heart problems probably were the result of a lifetime of untreated sleep apnea. If sleep apnea is treated correctly, these medical problems can be prevented, and even reversed. The sooner treatment is begun, the better the results.

Mr. Allen's story is dramatic. Not every case of long-term sleep apnea is so severe, and not every recovery is so striking. But in many ways Mr. Allen's story is typical — the snoring, the sleepiness, the fatigue, the loss of vigor, the threatening progress of an unidentified disease, the frustrations of seeking help where none seems available.

Most sleep apnea sufferers have followed a similar path. Today, more than six years after publication of the first edition of this book, the public and the medical community finally are becoming more aware of the signs, symptoms, and seriousness of sleep apnea. In addition, sleep specialists have learned more about the diagnosis and treatment of sleep apnea and other forms of sleep-disordered breathing.

As knowledge and awareness increase, and as more accredited sleep disorders centers are available, one must hope that people are more likely to be diagnosed at an earlier stage and can begin treatment before they develop severe medical complications.

What Are the Symptoms of Sleep Apnea and Sleep-Disordered Breathing?

If you have a sleep disorder, you may be the last person to recognize the symptoms. After all, you are asleep when many of them occur. Often it is a friend or loved one who notices that someone's sleep, or his breathing during sleep, is not quite normal.

So, husbands, wives, children, and friends: See if the 10 most common symptoms of sleep apnea and sleep-disordered breathing are familiar to you.

The first two symptoms go together.

Symptoms 1 and 2

LOUD, IRREGULAR SNORING, SNORTS, GASPS, AND OTHER UNUSUAL BREATHING SOUNDS DURING SLEEP

The most obvious sign of sleep apnea is very noisy snoring that stops and starts in an unrhythmic manner during the night. The snoring stops when the person stops breathing. It begins again, sometimes with a snort or a gasp, when the person takes the next breath.

Irregular snoring, with breathing that stops, is different from the quiet, relaxed sawing of ZZZs that most of us do occasionally, especially if we're sleeping on our back. Apnea-type snoring is noisy, labored, and sometimes explosive, and strongly suggests some struggle or discomfort on the part of the snorer.

Another characteristic of severe apnea-type snoring is that the snorer seems to snore in almost any position. Rolling over on the side often does not help, as it usually does in the case of simple, harmless nonapnea snoring. Some patients, however, snore and have apnea only when sleeping on their back.

Heavy or labored breathing, without snoring, can be a sign of sleep-disordered breathing that is a close relative of sleep apnea and also needs medical attention.

Symptom 3

PAUSES IN BREATHING DURING SLEEP

Everyone's breathing is irregular at certain times during sleep. For example, your breathing may pause for a moment just as you fall asleep or as you awaken. During periods of dreaming, breathing tends to speed up and slow down in an irregular manner. These are all normal changes in breathing while asleep.

However, a person with sleep apnea frequently stops breathing entirely and may hold his breath for a surprisingly long time. Each of these periods during which breathing has stopped is called an apnea episode, or an apnea event. An apnea event may last from 10 seconds to more than a minute.

Sleep specialists measure sleep apnea in several ways. One is to count the number of apnea events during the night and measure how long they last. A person is considered to have signs of sleep apnea if he stops breathing for more than 10 seconds at a time and if this happens more than five times during an hour of sleep. This would be a very mild case of sleep apnea, but one that would bear watching to ensure that it did not become worse.

Apnea events do not happen just once or twice, but 5, 10, 20, or more times per hour. In some people, apnea may occur only while lying on the back or only during certain stages of sleep. In other people, it can continue all night in all positions.

By morning a person with sleep apnea may have experienced hundreds of fairly long periods of nonbreathing. One might think that a person would be aware of such a struggle to breathe during sleep. Some apnea patients do notice that they awaken briefly with a snort, particularly during naps or when they nod off in a sitting position. A few people with sleep apnea will wake up completely to breathe, but usually they don't know why they have awakened. They are likely to describe their problem as "insomnia."

However, most people with sleep apnea are unaware of having a sleep/breathing problem. Many have absolutely no complaints about their sleep. They believe they sleep "just fine," and only wish their bedmate would stop bothering them about their snoring.

A tape recording of a person's sleeping sounds can be useful for convincing both that person and his doctor that he suffers from a breathing disorder during sleep.

Symptoms 4 and 5

EXCESSIVE DAYTIME SLEEPINESS AND/OR FATIGUE

The most common sleep complaint of people with sleep apnea is that they get "too much sleep." Sleep specialists call this symptom excessive daytime sleepiness (EDS).

Two-thirds of sleep apnea patients suffer from some degree of EDS, and they may not even know it. People often have simply lived with the effects of sleep apnea for so long, or it has crept up on them so gradually, that they do not know what "normal" feels like. They may think that they feel normal, that drowsiness is just a sign of getting older, or that maybe they just need a vacation.

However, it is not normal to have to fight to stay awake at your desk at work, at the wheel while driving, at the dinner table, at parties, at sporting events. If you are struggling against sleepiness during the day, you need to find out what is causing your abnormal drowsiness. Find out now before it further undermines your life.

Excessive daytime sleepiness results mainly from poor nighttime sleep; in sleep apnea, the person's sleep is interrupted throughout the night by repeated apnea events. He does not get enough sleep, and his sleep is of poor quality. As a result of these sleep/breathing disturbances, someone with sleep apnea builds up a "sleep debt" — an ongoing need for sleep that carries over into his daytime life. His sleep debt pressures him to fall asleep easily and frequently during the daytime — at his desk at work, while reading or watching TV, while driving.

Fatigue is another common problem for people with sleep apnea. Fatigue is different from sleepiness. Rather than a desire to go to sleep, fatigue is a sense of feeling exhausted, drained. People with sleep apnea typically feel fatigued a lot of the time. Often, because their apnea has been present for years and has gotten progressively worse, they are not even aware that they are more tired than normal. Or they assume that their fatigue is simply a normal sign of aging.

Again, as with drowsiness, a constant feeling of exhaustion is not normal. It is not an inevitable sign of age. A person who feels fatigued a lot of the time probably has a medical problem. It may or may not be sleep apnea. But a physician should certainly consider sleep apnea as a possible cause of unexplained fatigue and refer a chronically fatigued patient to a sleep clinic for testing if he has suspicious symptoms.

CASE STUDY

Mr. Bell's wife pleaded with him to see a doctor about his gasping and irregular breathing during sleep. But Mr. Bell was in excellent physical condition and at the age of 46 could outrun much younger men in 10 kilometer races. He had seen a TV show about sleep problems and knew that some apnea and snoring can be normal, so he ignored his wife's request.

A life insurance company reviewed Mr. Bell's medical records and noticed that the doctor's note suggested "possible sleep apnea," so they denied him insurance. Mr. Bell went to a sleep center, hoping to prove he was in perfect health. Instead he learned that, in fact, he had moderately severe apnea.

Mr. Bell received treatment for his sleep apnea, and a follow-up study of his sleep showed an excellent response. His insurance application was approved, which pleased him; in addition, Mr. Bell realized that he felt much better. He was amazed that he had not noticed the signs of sleep apnea before treatment.

The moral of Mr. Bell's story is clear: if your bedmate is concerned that you have sleep apnea, he or she may be right, even if you don't feel ill. Some people can tolerate very significant amounts of sleep apnea without being aware of it. Apparently they do not notice a deterioration in the quality of their sleep or their daytime alertness, nor are they bothered by "insomnia" or fatigue. Mr. Bell is typical of former sleep apnea patients after treatment — they are astonished at feeling so much more wide-awake, energetic, and alive.

Symptom 6

OBESITY

Obesity is fairly common among people with sleep apnea. A complicated relationship exists between weight and sleep apnea: sleep apnea makes the weight problem worse, and vice versa. Losing weight usually helps the sleep apnea, but people often cannot lose weight until after the sleep apnea has been treated. The sleep apnea–obesity relationship is described in more detail in Chapter 8.

Not everyone who is overweight suffers from sleep apnea, nor is everyone who has sleep apnea necessarily overweight. In fact, individuals who are quite thin can have severe sleep apnea.

CASE STUDY

Mr. Johnson was a 29-year-old who snored badly and had been tired "for years." His wife had noticed pauses in his breathing during sleep, but they were infrequent, and she was a good sleeper, so she didn't mind his snoring.

Several doctors over several years had performed thorough medical examinations and had concluded that stress or underlying depression was the likely cause of Mr. Johnson's chronic tiredness. During his last evaluation he mentioned the snoring and the apnea that his wife had observed, but he was told he was "too young and too thin" to have any trouble with sleep apnea. Mr. Johnson eventually was studied in a sleep center, and it was discovered that he stopped breathing 43 times an hour. With treatment using nasal CPAP (see Chapter 7), Mr. Johnson's fatigue disappeared entirely.

Symptom 7

CHANGES IN ALERTNESS, MEMORY, PERSONALITY, OR BEHAVIOR

Sleep apnea can mimic depression, laziness, or personality change. Increased irritability, shortness of temper, or "crabbiness" are very often caused by sleep apnea but may be explained away as the result of stress in the person's life.

As with the other symptoms of sleep apnea, family and friends often are the first to notice behavioral signs of sleep apnea. These changes in behavior can include a gradual shift in sleeping or napping habits, in the person's energy level, in his productivity at home or at work, or in his mood or disposition. Any of these changes in behavior, which the person himself might not notice, may suggest sleep apnea.

CASE STUDY

Mr. Arnold was under a lot of stress. His business was in trouble from new competition. His wife was drinking heavily, and their marriage seemed to be breaking down. His business partner was concerned that he was gaining weight, seemed irritable and depressed, and was not his usual outgoing self with the office staff and customers. Mr. Arnold was distractible in business meetings, and his once photographic memory for business statistics was slipping badly.

His partner suggested that he see a psychologist and get help to deal with his stress, depression, and marital problems. He took his partner's advice. But counseling did not help, and his family doctor referred him to a psychiatrist. The psychiatrist noted his snoring and sleepiness and sent him for testing at a sleep center, where he was found to be suffering from sleep apnea. Treatment resolved his personality change, memory problems, and poor work performance.

Unexplained changes in mental sharpness or in personality should arouse a suspicion of possible sleep apnea, particularly if these changes are accompanied by apnea during sleep, fatigue, weight gain, or other symptoms mentioned in this chapter.

Other Symptoms of Sleep Apnea (Symptoms 8, 9, and 10)

Other symptoms sometimes associated with sleep apnea include the following:

- Impotence
- Morning headaches
- Bed-wetting

Few people have all the symptoms of sleep apnea. Most people show only one or two obvious signs of the disorder.

It is important to emphasize that any of the symptoms of sleep apnea might also be caused by other, possibly harmful conditions. For this and other reasons, a person suspected of having sleep apnea or any other type of sleep-disordered breathing should be tested by a physician who specializes in sleep disorders so that other disorders can be ruled out and the correct diagnosis made.

s u m m a r y

A person shows signs of sleep apnea syndrome that may affect his health:

- If he stops breathing for more than 10 seconds at a time, and
- If this happens more than five times during an hour of sleep.

The following are the most common signs and symptoms of sleep apnea:

1. Loud, irregular snoring
2. Snorts, gasps, and other unusual breathing sounds during sleep
3. Long pauses in breathing during sleep
4. Excessive daytime sleepiness

5. Fatigue
6. Obesity
7. Changes in alertness, memory, personality, or behavior
8. Impotence
9. Morning headaches
10. Bed-wetting

If you have loud, irregular snoring or labored breathing during sleep plus any of the other preceding symptoms, you should ask your doctor to refer you to an accredited sleep center for evaluation.

chapter 2

Sleep Apnea Harms Health and Home Life

People with sleep apnea pay a high price over the years. They suffer significant damage from the poor quality of their sleep, from their nightly struggle to breathe, and from the lower than normal oxygen supply in their blood during the night. The family, friends, employers, and business associates of people with untreated sleep apnea also pay a high price because of negative changes in personality, decreased work performance, and overall diminished ability to fulfill their social and emotional responsibilities.

The long-term damage from sleep apnea can be divided into health effects and social and psychological effects. The seriousness of the damage depends on how long the apnea has been present and the person's overall health.

*H*ealth Effects of Sleep Apnea

Most of the serious health problems from sleep apnea develop gradually over the long term. But one source of injury is very abrupt — the auto wreck.

Automobile Accidents

Automobile accidents are three times more common among people with untreated sleep apnea than in normal people. Nearly 20 percent of sleep apnea patients admit to having had auto accidents from falling asleep at the wheel.[1] Recent studies of long-haul truck drivers have found that nearly half of them had obvious symptoms of sleep apnea.[2] In 1996 the American Medical Association urged physicians to learn about sleep disorders and to warn their patients of the dangers of driving and working while fatigued or sleepy.[3]

Sleepiness while driving usually develops gradually over weeks or months. Before having an actual auto accident, most if not all apnea patients have had very brief "micro-sleeps" while driving. They nod off for an instant, perhaps also experiencing a prolonged eye blink or an actual bobbing of the head. This brief sleep may result in the car wandering in the lane, drifting onto the shoulder, or even crossing into the next lane.

The driver may not notice, or may ignore or not admit, the warning signal of a potentially life-threatening episode of sleepiness. The family of a person with life-threatening sleepiness may have observed him repeatedly falling asleep, even on short trips; yet the driver may absolutely deny that he is sleepy or dangerous.

The reasons for denial can be complicated, ranging from lack of awareness to pride to unconscious denial of the problem. One study compared the accident records of men and women with untreated sleep apnea. Men were about four times more likely than women to drive while sleepy and to have auto accidents.[4]

Auto accidents among people with sleep apnea are so common that some sleep clinics give each sleep apnea patient a letter advising him not to drive until he has received treatment. Accidents in the workplace can also be a major risk for people with sleep apnea and for their coworkers and clients. In the transportation industry, untreated sleep apnea is a public danger when it affects school bus drivers, airplane and ship pilots, railroad engineers, truck drivers, heavy equipment operators, and carpool drivers. People in these occupations who ever experience drowsiness on the job have an obligation either to identify and treat the cause of their drowsiness or to change occupations.

Once treatment for sleep apnea has begun, it is important for both health and safety to make sure that the treatment is actually having an effect. *Feeling* cured is not the same as *being* cured, as the following case illustrates.

CASE STUDY

Mr. Rodgers was diagnosed with moderately severe obstructive sleep apnea and underwent UPPP (uvulopalatopharyngoplasty) surgery [discussed in Chapter 7]. His snoring disappeared, he felt better, and he no longer fell asleep at the wrong times. The surgeon recommended that he return to the sleep center for a retest to see how much improvement had actually been achieved by the surgery. Mr. Rodgers refused to be retested because he was "absolutely sure" he was cured.

Six months later Mr. Rodgers fell asleep while driving and wrecked his car. In retrospect, he could recall occasionally feeling drowsy even though he had improved significantly after surgery. A follow-up sleep study showed that he still had 50 percent of his sleep apnea. Further treatment resulted in full control of his symptoms.

If you suffer from excessive drowsiness, you owe it to yourself, your family, and others on the highway to refrain from driving until you have been tested to determine the cause of your problem and have begun effective treatment.

Breathing, Circulation, and Heart Problems

The cardiovascular (heart and circulatory system) and pulmonary (lung) effects of sleep apnea are very serious; over a period of years these effects become life-threatening. Strokes are three times more common in heavy snorers than in nonsnorers,[5] and heart attack is more than 20 times more likely in people with untreated sleep apnea.[6] The cardiovascular effects of sleep apnea result in the nocturnal sudden death of approximately 2,000 to 3,000 people per year in the United States.[7] Let's look at some of the ways in which sleep apnea can damage people's health.

Low blood oxygen concentration during the night is typical in a person with sleep apnea. This is responsible for much of the long-term harm resulting from sleep apnea. With each apnea event, the blood oxygen drops to an abnormally low level, depriving the body's cells of oxygen. The brain is particularly susceptible to low oxygen. If the low blood oxygen is severe and continues over a long period, it can unfavorably affect the brain. This may explain the changes in personality, memory, alertness, and coordination seen in people with sleep apnea.[8]

High blood pressure is one important cardiovascular effect of low blood oxygen. High blood pressure is seen in 35 percent to 50 percent of sleep apnea patients. Chronic high blood pressure results in enlargement of the heart, which is a risk factor for stroke and heart failure.[9]

The relationship between high blood pressure and sleep apnea is complicated and not well understood. Some people have significant improvement in their blood pressure once their sleep apnea is treated. Other people show little change because their high blood pressure has other causes.

Blood pressure may be indirectly improved when the treatment of sleep apnea allows the patient to lose weight and enjoy regular exercise. Excess weight contributes to high blood pressure, and regular exercise can help to lower blood pressure.

Patients on high doses of blood pressure medications should make sure their doctors follow them carefully after their sleep apnea is treated to see if they need less medication. Otherwise they may develop symptoms of low blood pressure because their body no longer needs so much medication. Careful adjustments of medications are necessary.

Sleep apnea contributes notably to a particular type of high blood pressure: unusually high pressure in the artery that carries blood from the right side of the heart to the lungs. This occurs mainly in people who have other health problems and already have low blood oxygen when they are awake. In time this condition can lead to enlargement of the right side of the heart and fluid congestion in the lungs.[9-12]

Arrhythmia (abnormal heart rhythm) is seen in more than 90 percent of sleep apnea patients.[12] Abnormal slowing of the heart, long pauses (more than two seconds), extra beats, and several other types of arrhythmias are associated with sleep apnea. People with sleep apnea are thought to run a higher than normal risk of sudden death from heart failure during the night, probably because of a fatal arrhythmia.[13]

The **operation of the lungs** is affected by changes in blood pressure (described earlier) that result from low blood oxygen. In addition, the low oxygen and high carbon dioxide concentrations in the blood result in abnormal blood chemistry. These changes in blood chemistry also disturb the functioning of the lungs.[14]

The combined damage from cardiopulmonary disturbances — abnormal blood pressure relationships in the heart and lungs, abnormal blood chemistry from too much carbon dioxide and too little oxygen, arrhythmias — is thought by most sleep specialists to be the greatest long-term danger to health from sleep apnea.[15]

*S*ocial and Psychological Effects

The fatigue, sleepiness, and medical complications that result from sleep apnea can virtually destroy a person's life.

Work performance is often profoundly undermined. People with sleep apnea may miss work frequently, arrive at work late, become drowsy or fall asleep at work, and suffer from poor concentration, memory loss, and poor job performance. Their bosses and colleagues seldom understand their problems and often assume that the unusual behavior is due to drugs, alcohol, or serious personality problems. Promotions are missed, jobs are lost, and promising careers are sidetracked.

Home life and social life also suffer. Studies have shown that married people with sleep apnea tend to become socially isolated and alienated from their partners and children. The fatigue and sleepiness of the sleep apnea sufferer lead him to participate less and less in family activities and relationships and to spend more and more time withdrawn or sleeping. Family life often begins to feel more like a burden than a source of support.[16]

His family may become critical of his inactivity, decreased work around the house, or negative and crabby attitude. The result is a puzzled, resentful, increasingly uncommunicative family. These problems may contribute to marital conflicts, child-raising difficulties, and divorce.

Psychological and memory problems are frequent results of sleep apnea. **Irritability** is common in people with moderate to severe sleep apnea, as are other personality changes, such as depression, and, less commonly, **memory impairment, confusion, anger,** and even **physical abuse. Loss of alertness and concentration** are not unusual. Patients with sleep apnea score lower than normal on tests for attention and concentration and on other tests of brain activity.[8]

The loss of mental acuity usually is so gradual that the person may not realize it is happening. First he may find that reading is a chore, so he will read less. Then he may have trouble concentrating on other tasks or remembering words. It may not be until after his sleep apnea is under treatment and his mental facility begins to return that he realizes how much he has lost.

These neurologic changes are due to both poor sleep and the abnormally low oxygen levels in the blood during sleep (discussed previously).

To summarize, driving accidents may be the most immediate threat of death from sleep apnea. In the longer term, sleep apnea leads to life-threatening medical complications and psychological and social difficulties. Most of these consequences can be lessened or eliminated with treatment of the apnea. Treatment is discussed in Chapter 7.

*D*iagnosing and Treating Sleep Apnea

Who Suffers from Sleep Apnea?

When does a person's tendency toward sleep apnea first arise? This is difficult to pinpoint because sleep apnea results from the combination of several risk factors.

Sleep apnea can be found at all ages. In some people the tendency may be present at birth. Sleep apnea may be the later stage of a breathing disorder that begins early in life as a slight breathing abnormality — some part of the automatic breathing reflex that is slightly irregular.

A breathing abnormality is more likely to develop into sleep apnea when other important risk factors are present: obesity; an insensitive breathing reflex (see Chapter 3); a slight failure in coordination between the breathing muscles; an upper airway that is narrowed or obstructed by blockages in the nasal passages, large tonsils or adenoids, a large tongue, or a short lower jaw; and so on. Any of these factors may combine so that a slight breathing instability in a young person gradually evolves into a permanent abnormality in sleep breathing in an adult.[17]

The tendency to develop sleep apnea is probably inherited in some people. For example, a person may inherit an airway whose shape is easily obstructed. Or he may inherit a weak breathing response to carbon dioxide. Either one or a combination of several inherited factors may set the stage for a person to develop sleep apnea.[18]

Sex is a factor in the development of sleep apnea. Men are about three times more likely to have sleep apnea than women.[19] The reasons for this difference are unclear, but they may have to do with sexual differences in the structure of the airway or in muscle tone. The effects of sex hormones may also be a factor (e.g., progesterone in women versus testosterone in men). Body weight is another factor. Obese people suffer a much higher incidence of sleep apnea than people of ideal weight (see Chapter 8).

In terms of age, sleep apnea is primarily a condition of middle age or older. This is true for several reasons. First, with age there is a loss of muscle tone in the throat during sleep. Second, when people do have untreated sleep apnea, the condition becomes worse as they grow older. Third, body weight tends to increase with age, often beginning after age 40. By the time the symptoms of sleep apnea are serious enough to attract medical attention, the person may be in his 40s or 50s and may be suffering from obesity, pulmonary complications, arrhythmia, or even congestive heart failure. The average age of patients in one sleep clinic was reported to be 52.[20]

However, sleep apnea can occur at any age. Children can develop sleep apnea. In fact, now that tonsillectomies are less common than they used to be, sleep apnea is probably more prevalent in children than it was a generation ago. Children who have enlarged tonsils or adenoids or who are obese are the most likely to develop sleep apnea. [See Chapter 9 for information about apnea in infants and about sudden infant death syndrome (SIDS) and Chapter 10 for more about sleep apnea in older children.]

A number of drugs aggravate sleep apnea. These include alcohol, sedatives, hypnotic drugs ("sleeping pills"), and some heart medications (short-acting beta blockers, such as propranolol) (see the Appendix).

Why Haven't You Heard of Sleep Apnea Before?

It has been estimated that 20 million Americans may have sleep apnea.[21] Among 30- to 60-year-olds, one of every four men and one of every 10 women show some signs of sleep apnea. In a study of industrial workers in Israel, one of every five was classified as having some degree of sleep apnea.[22] These are surprisingly large numbers of people, considering that a few years ago hardly anybody had ever heard of sleep apnea.

So if sleep apnea is this common, why haven't you heard about it before? The answer is that sleep apnea has always been around, but it was not recognized by the medical community until recently.

One of the earliest descriptions of sleep apnea was published in 1877 by an observant medical man named W. H. Broadbent. He did not call the condition sleep apnea, but he described the two major types of apnea that today are called obstructive apnea and central apnea.

During the late 1800s several additional reports were published about patients who suffered from abnormal daytime sleepiness and had difficulty breathing while asleep. In 1890 an early American neurologist and toxicologist named Silas Weir Mitchell wrote the first detailed accounts of a breathing disorder that occurred during sleep and began to unravel the mystery of what causes sleep apnea.

Unfortunately for those suffering from sleep apnea, bacteria came into vogue soon after that. Medical attention focused on sleep diseases that were caused by microbes, such as sleeping sickness, and little interest or credence was given to other kinds of sleep disorders or their causes. As a result, much of what had been learned or suggested about sleep disorders lapsed into neglect.

It was not until the 1950s that several groups of scientists began to make careful observations of actual sleeping people. They developed an electronic technique for measuring and studying sleep, called polysomnography (see Chapter 6). Using this technique, they began to discover interesting things about what goes on during sleep. They learned, for example, that sleep is not at all a time of peaceful inactivity. This unexpected discovery stimulated an explosion of interest in sleep research and intensified the quest for a better understanding of sleep, both normal and abnormal.

It soon became apparent that events during sleep can profoundly affect a person's health. As explained by Dr. William Dement, one of the leaders in this field, "It is possible for individuals to be entirely normal awake and deathly ill asleep."[23] Thus a new field of medicine — sleep disorders medicine — began to take shape.

In the past 15 years sleep researchers have learned how to recognize the signs of various abnormal sleep conditions — sleep apnea and other forms of sleep-disordered breathing, narcolepsy, nocturnal myoclonus, idiopathic central nervous system hypersomnolence, and others — that previously had been difficult or impossible to diagnose. Physicians are becoming better informed and are beginning to diagnose sleep apnea in patients who previously might simply have been treated for insomnia, heart problems, or some other symptom.

Confirming the Diagnosis and Treating Sleep Apnea

Once you have been given a tentative diagnosis of sleep apnea or a similar sleep/breathing disorder, an all-night sleep test should be arranged. Proper testing for sleep disorders is important because several sleep disorders have superficial similarities and might be confused with sleep apnea or be incorrectly diagnosed if testing is not done properly. An incorrect diagnosis, leading to incorrect treatment, can be a serious error. For example, medications that are often prescribed for narcolepsy or insomnia can actually worsen sleep apnea, so a correct diagnosis is very important.

Narcolepsy is a sleep disorder in which people have irresistible "sleep attacks" at inappropriate times, somewhat as in sleep apnea. However, narcolepsy is a distinct neurologic disorder with its own characteristic symptoms (cataplexy, sleep paralysis, and hypnagogic hallucinations) not found in sleep apnea.

Insomnia is sometimes confused with sleep apnea. Insomnia has numerous causes, and only a few people who have insomnia also have sleep apnea.

Two other sleep disorders sometimes occur alone or along with sleep apnea. These are periodic limb movement in sleep (PLMS, also called periodic leg movement disorder, PLMD, or nocturnal myoclonus) and restless leg syndrome (RLS). Again, appropriate testing by an experienced sleep disorders specialist will avoid confusing one sleep disorder with another.

An overnight sleep test will:

- Confirm whether you actually have sleep apnea or another form of sleep-disordered breathing
- Determine the type of sleep/breathing disorder, which must be known in order to select the appropriate treatment
- Rule out other sleep disorders

Chapters 4 through 7 of this book will take you through the processes of diagnosis and treatment of sleep apnea. Chapter 4 describes the three types of sleep apnea. Chapter 5 discusses some of the difficulties in diagnosing sleep apnea. Testing for sleep apnea is described in Chapter 6. Treatment choices are discussed in Chapter 7.

Chapter 3 is included for those readers who would like a better understanding of sleep and the causes of sleep apnea.

summary

- Sleep apnea is not yet widely recognized by family doctors.

- Sleep apnea can occur at any age but is most common in middle age, particularly among men and obese people.

- Sleep apnea is treatable.

- Sleep apnea can devastate a person's career, wreak havoc on family and social life, and cause psychological and memory problems.

- Sleep apnea can be life-threatening if not treated. It results in:
Auto accidents
Workplace accidents
Abnormal blood chemistry
High blood pressure
Arrhythmia (irregular heartbeat)
Other heart complications
Lung complications
Loss of alertness, memory, concentration
Death

Normal Sleep, Snoring, and the Development of Sleep Apnea

*T*his chapter is for the reader who likes to understand how things work. Not everyone will be interested in finding out what happens inside his or her body to cause sleep apnea. But anyone can understand the causes of sleep apnea, and that understanding will help make it seem less frightening or mysterious.

Understanding the cause of sleep apnea will also give you a better grasp of the kinds of treatment that are used and of the importance of carrying through with long-term treatment. You will be better equipped to discuss treatment options with your doctor and to play an active role in choosing the most appropriate treatment.

*S*leep — Normal and Abnormal

To understand the causes and results of sleep apnea, it helps to know a little about what happens during a normal night's sleep.

Why Do We Sleep?

Nobody knows exactly why we sleep. At one time people thought that sleep was just a rest period for our brains. Then polysomnography was developed. This technology allows scientists to make electrical recordings of brain activities during sleep. Scientists were surprised to discover that brains are anything but idle during the night.

Some theories suggest that we sleep to overcome body fatigue. Our bodies do seem to overcome fatigue during sleep, but studies have shown that it is our brain, not our muscles, that requires sleep in order to feel rested and function normally.

How much sleep do we need? Actually there is no "normal" amount of sleep that is right for everybody. The amount of sleep a person needs is a very individual matter and also varies according to age and circumstances (Figure 3.1).

It used to be said, for example, that babies needed 21 hours of sleep per day, but now it is known that the amount of sleep they need varies a great deal from infant to infant. Sixteen-year-olds seem to need approximately 10 or 11 hours, and this decreases to about eight hours for an average adult. There are cases of healthy, alert adults who do fine on four hours of sleep, but that is rare. The record for habitually short sleep seems to be about three hours per night.[1] No one has ever been documented to need no sleep.

What happens if people are experimentally deprived of sleep for several days? Sleep deprivation upsets the body's physiologic systems: hormones, immune system, blood pressure regulation, digestive system, and urine production. Normally our physiologic processes go through 24-hour ups and downs. Sleeping and waking up in the morning are signals that our biological clock uses to keep those physiologic systems synchronized with each other. A person who is not sleeping well or whose sleep schedule is irregular (for example, because of shift work) does not have normal signals to reset his clock each day and keep things running smoothly. This may help to explain why disturbances of the digestive system, headaches, and other illnesses are more common in people who do shift work.

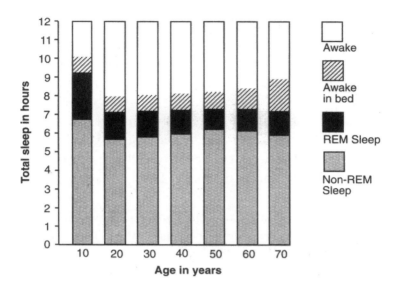

Figure 3.1
Changes in sleep over a lifetime.

In terms of behavior, sleep-deprived people have periodic bouts of drowsiness when their built-in biological clock tries to get them to go to sleep. They suffer a gradual, increasing loss of the ability to concentrate, and their ability to think becomes dull. These effects on thinking and memory are especially damaging in school-aged children and teenagers, many of whom are seriously sleep-deprived.[2]

Sleep-deprived people also may become irritable and disoriented, and may have dreamlike hallucinations. Reactions become slow and erratic. In a sleep-deprived driver, this condition commonly leads to auto accidents. Research shows that even as many as seven hours of sleep for seven nights in a row can slow a person's reaction time and interfere with tasks such as driving. Nine hours of sleep are needed, consistently every night, for reaction time to be at its best.[3]

In itself, sleep deprivation is not fatal. However, it certainly causes fatalities when it interferes with a person's ability to perform normally. When a long-haul truck driver falls asleep at the wheel and crashes, an average of four innocent victims die with him.

To be at our best, each of us needs a certain quantity of sleep every night. If we do not get enough sleep, we tend to build up a sleep "debt." This leads to a tendency to feel drowsy during the day and to fall asleep more readily.

But the *quantity* of sleep we get is not the whole story. Equally important is the *quality* of our sleep. Does it come in large, continuous blocks, or is it fragmented into short naps? Do we get enough "deep" sleep?

The quality of our sleep is related to a series of sleep stages that the brain passes through during the night. These are described in the next section.

In people with sleep apnea, sleep is broken up by numerous awakenings during the night, reducing the quantity of sleep they obtain. In addition, the numerous awakenings break up the structure, or continuity, of their sleep. They miss out on some of the normal stages of sleep. This lowers the quality of their sleep. Thus sleep apnea affects both the quantity and the quality of sleep. Let's look a little more closely at what goes on in your brain while you are sleeping.

The Stages of Normal Sleep

After you go to sleep, the activities of your brain and body settle into fairly predictable patterns. Sleep researchers have discovered that there are two kinds of sleep: REM sleep and non-REM (or NREM) sleep. REM stands for rapid eye movement, and in a moment you will see why. REM and NREM sleep alternate with each other during the night.

NREM sleep is "quiet" sleep. Your breathing and brain activity are slow and regular, and your body is quiet and relaxed. You may dream, but the dreams will be more thoughtlike than emotional.

REM sleep, in contrast, is "active" sleep. There are active changes in your physiology during REM sleep. For example, your breathing becomes irregular, alternating between slow and fast. You may stop breathing every now and then for several seconds. Your body temperature rises, and the blood circulation in your brain increases. The large muscles of your body — your leg and arm muscles — actually become paralyzed: you cannot move them, except for little twitches of your face and fingertips. But your eye muscles become very active and move your eyes back and forth as if they were watching a ping-pong match. This, of course, is the rapid eye movement that led to the term *REM sleep.* Much, but not all, of your dreaming occurs during REM sleep. The most vivid, intense, emotional dreams almost always occur during REM sleep.

A typical night's sleep begins with "quiet" NREM sleep. There are four stages of NREM sleep, which progress from light to heavy sleep. Then, rather abruptly, about 70 to 90 minutes from the beginning of sleep, your sleep lightens from its deepest level to reach the first "active" REM period. That first REM sleep period usually lasts about 10 minutes. It ends when sleep shifts back into lighter stage 2 NREM sleep. Then sleep begins to deepen and the cycle starts all over again.

This cycle takes about 90 minutes and repeats itself throughout the night. Early in the night, the REM periods in the cycle are shorter. During the second half of the night, REM periods become longer, sometimes as long as 60 minutes, separated only by short periods of stage 2 NREM sleep (Figure 3.2).

The total amount of REM sleep during the night varies with age. Newborn babies spend about half of their sleeping time in REM sleep. By adulthood REM sleep has decreased to about one quarter of our total sleep time.

We all seem to need REM sleep, although nobody knows exactly why. The need may be related to REM dreaming, during which we seem to "process" the emotion-laden experiences of waking life.

In any case, our bodies appear to have an automatic mechanism that "tries" to obtain the normal amount of REM sleep for us. When people are deprived of REM sleep and then allowed to sleep normally, they usually experience several nights of what is called REM rebound, in which they spend an especially long time in REM sleep. They often remember dreaming more and having more vivid and often scarier dreams than normal. It is as if their bodies sense that they have been deprived of REM sleep and are catching up on what was missed.

As you will see later in this chapter, people with sleep apnea are often deprived of the normal amount of REM sleep.

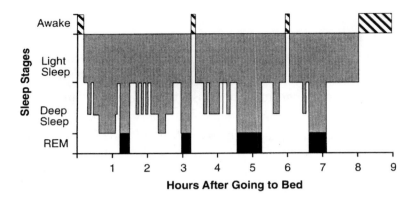

Figure 3.2

A typical night's sleep of a normal young adult. Notice how the sleep pattern shifts from stage to stage during the night.

Normal Breathing During Sleep

BREATHING CENTERS AND REFLEXES

Your breathing movements during sleep are controlled by automatic reflexes. These reflexes are driven by nerve sensors, which constantly monitor the chemistry of your blood and send signals to the breathing centers of your brain. These centers, in turn, send signals to your breathing muscles to regulate how fast and how powerfully you need to breathe at any particular time (Figure 3.3). This regulatory activity by the brain's breathing centers is one of the factors in the development of sleep apnea.

SENSORS AND "SET POINTS"

One group of nerve sensors for monitoring your blood chemistry is in your carotid bodies, which are located in the carotid arteries in your neck. They sense the amount of oxygen in the blood that is on its way to your brain and respond to low levels of oxygen in your blood. But even though oxygen is essential for life, particularly for your brain cells, these sensors are not the most important ones for your breathing reflex.

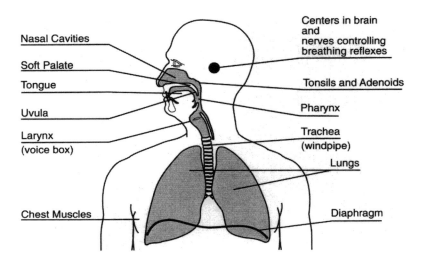

Figure 3.3
The parts of the body that are involved in the breathing reflex.

A more powerful set of sensors is in a deep and primitive part of your brain called the medulla. These sensors detect increases in the carbon dioxide in your cerebrospinal fluid (the fluid that bathes your brain and spinal cord). Carbon dioxide, your body's waste gas, is produced as the oxygen in your body is used up. A high concentration of carbon dioxide in your cerebrospinal fluid signals that your body needs to breathe. When you breathe, you exhale carbon dioxide and immediately inhale fresh oxygen.

The particular concentration of carbon dioxide that triggers these sensors can be called the "set point." Whenever the carbon dioxide concentration rises high enough to reach the set point, the breathing reflex is activated. The oxygen sensors probably work in a similar way, but their set points are not nearly as sensitive during sleep.

The set points that trigger your breathing reflexes can move up and down, depending on a number of factors, including whether you are awake or asleep. During sleep the set points do not have to be as sensitive to low oxygen and high carbon dioxide as they do when you are awake because your sleeping body needs less oxygen, your breathing is more shallow, and the air in your lungs is exchanged less vigorously. So as you pass from waking to sleeping to waking, the set points cycle up and down.[4]

Even during sleep the set points seem to change. For example, during REM sleep the breathing responses become less sensitive. More carbon dioxide is tolerated, and the oxygen concentration can sometimes drop extremely low during REM sleep before the breathing reflexes finally are triggered.[4] The sensitivity of the set points is another factor in the development of sleep apnea.

BREATHING MUSCLES

The movements of breathing require the use of muscle groups in a number of places: the diaphragm, the rib cage (the intercostal and other muscles that attach to the ribs), the soft palate, the tongue, the upper and lower pharynx (the throat area behind the mouth), and the larynx (voice box). When breathing is normal, the actions of these assorted muscles are carefully coordinated. For example, when you inhale, your rib muscles contract, your tongue muscles automatically stabilize the position of your tongue, and your soft palate muscles become taut to hold your airway open. The coordination among these various muscle groups during breathing is another factor in the development of sleep apnea (Figure 3.4).

Snoring

Snoring occurs when your soft palate (the back part of the roof of your mouth) vibrates. A number of factors cause this. The muscle tone in your tongue and soft palate tends to decrease during sleep. They become more relaxed and can collapse together. This contributes to snoring. Other soft tissues, such as tonsils and tongue, can produce sounds that add to or change the quality of the snoring.

The position of the sleeper affects the amount of snoring. Lying on your back allows your tongue to fall back toward your throat and block your airway, so you are more likely to snore when you are lying on your back.

Anything that obstructs your airway will also contribute to snoring. For example, you are more likely to snore if you have large adenoids or

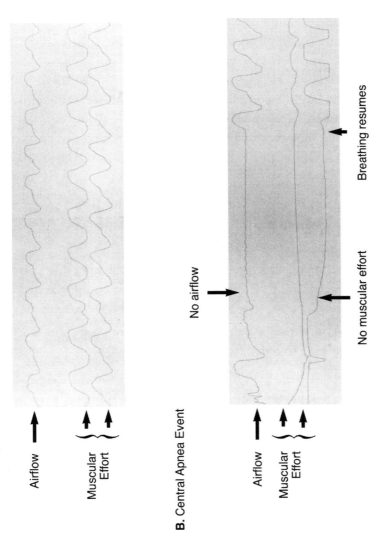

Figure 3.4

Typical patterns of breathing, showing airflow and movement of breathing muscles, (A) during normal sleep and (B) in a central apnea event, in which the breathing reflexes do not operate normally.

a large tongue or if your nasal passages are swollen from a cold or allergies.

Age is also a factor. Older people tend to snore more because muscle tone tends to decrease with age.

Other factors also aggravate snoring; alcoholic beverages, certain medications, and sheer physical exhaustion may be associated with heavy snoring.

Mere snoring, by itself, is not the same as sleep apnea. Many people snore without having the complete interruptions of breathing and sleep that are the signs of sleep apnea. Light or occasional snoring that does not interrupt breathing is not a health threat, although it can be a terrific annoyance to a sleeping partner. The solutions to harmless occasional snoring include the following:

- Sleep on your side. You can train yourself to sleep on your side using a sleep position monitor (see Chapter 7).
- Avoid alcohol before going to bed.
- Check with your doctor to see whether any medication you are taking (either by prescription or over the counter) may be aggravating the snoring (see Chapter 7 and the Appendix).
- If nasal congestion is a problem, ask your doctor about an antihistamine to reduce swelling.
- Decrease your body weight.
- The sleeping partner can wear soft foam earplugs when necessary. They are available from industrial safety stores.

When Simple Snoring Turns into Sleep Apnea

In some people the loss of muscle tone in the tongue and throat is accompanied by a number of other factors, discussed earlier in this chapter: an instability in the breathing reflexes, a structural narrowing of the airway, or a lack of coordination among the breathing muscles. Various types of sleep-disordered breathing can occur, ranging from mild to severe.

In some people slight or occasional snoring may gradually develop into the heavy, more violent snoring that indicates sleep apnea. This process often begins in adolescence with heavy snoring and occasional short clusters of apnea events. Gradually, the picture may change to heavier snoring with longer sequences of nonbreathing. Later in adulthood the pattern may evolve into obstructive apnea events that occur throughout nearly the whole night, with great disturbances in the structure of sleep, fluctuations in oxygen content of the blood, and daytime drowsiness.[5] In some older people who have never had trouble with sleep apnea, the loss of muscle tone that occurs with age is enough to trigger the development of sleep apnea.

The reason snoring may progress to sleep apnea in some people and not in others depends on the sum of all the factors we have described here: breathing reflexes, structure of the airway, muscle coordination, and inherited tendencies.

summary

- The most important aspects of sleep are:
  The quantity of sleep,
  The quality of sleep, and
  The amount of REM (rapid eye movement) sleep.

- Sleep apnea interferes with all three of these.

- An abnormality in the breathing reflex during sleep can contribute to the development of sleep apnea.

- Snoring is caused by loss of muscle tone in the tongue and throat.

- Most of the sounds of typical snoring are caused by the vibration of the soft palate.

- Snoring in which breathing does not stop probably is harmless. You may be able to decrease or eliminate this type of snoring by following suggestions in this chapter.

- Snoring in which breathing stops is a symptom of sleep apnea.

What Causes Sleep Apnea?

A Typical Mixed Apnea Event

C A S E   S T U D Y

Mr. Kennedy crawls into bed and turns out the light. He immediately falls asleep and begins to snore softly. His wife stuffs earplugs into her ears and wills herself to fall asleep quickly, before her husband really starts to snore. She reaches over and shakes his elbow.

"Roll over," she reminds him.

He complies, turns onto his side, and resumes his snoring.

Over the next few minutes the sound of each snore becomes louder, more prolonged, more emphatic. Then all at once the room is silent. The snoring has stopped.

Mr. Kennedy is lying very still. In fact, he is not breathing.

What has happened? The breathing center in Mr. Kennedy's brain has stopped working. As a result, the breathing muscles in his diaphragm and chest receive no signals. They stop moving. (This is a sign of central apnea.)

When breathing movements stop, oxygen cannot get into the lungs, nor can carbon dioxide get out. Consequently, the oxygen concentration in Mr. Kennedy's blood begins to drop and the concentration of carbon dioxide increases.

Mr. Kennedy is slowly suffocating.

Extreme concentrations of oxygen and carbon dioxide eventually stimulate his nerve sensors. (The farther their set point is from "normal," the longer it will take for this to happen. See Chapter 3.) When Mr. Kennedy's sensors finally respond, they tell his brain's breathing center to start working again. His breathing center again sends signals to the breathing muscles, and once again he begins to make breathing movements.

However, Mr. Kennedy's problems are not over; even though the chest muscles have begun to work, no air is going in or out of his lungs. This is because the airway in his throat collapsed shut when he first stopped breathing. His chest heaves in and out now, even shaking the mattress with the force of the muscle contractions; but his throat is closed, so there still is no actual movement of air in and out. (This is a sign of obstructive apnea.)

Mr. Kennedy may struggle for a breath of air for as long as a minute, or even longer. Meanwhile, the oxygen supply in his body is running out and the carbon dioxide is accumulating.

Fortunately for Mr. Kennedy and the rest of our species, we all have a primitive, fail-safe, emergency arousal response. It awakens us at just such times as this and keeps us from suffocating during sleep. When Mr. Kennedy's arousal response finally is triggered, he wakes up. His body jerks and he gasps for air with a series of loud, snorting breaths, sucking oxygen into his lungs like a diver returning from the depths. This is the explosive snoring that is typical of sleep apnea.

In just a few seconds fresh air pours into his lungs and the oxygen concentration in his blood reaches nearly normal, the carbon dioxide is expelled, and he returns to sleep. The arousal has been so brief that Mr. Kennedy is not aware of being awakened. But the normal pattern of his sleep has been broken. People with severe apnea may never reach deep sleep; they have very fragmented REM sleep because of the constant arousals. Thus throughout the night it is the deepest sleep that is most disturbed.

A short while after Mr. Kennedy returns to sleep — perhaps two minutes, perhaps five — the whole process will repeat itself.

Mr. Kennedy is an example of a person who has mixed apnea, a combination of central sleep apnea and obstructive sleep apnea.

The Three Types of Sleep Apnea

There are three kinds of sleep apnea, classified according to their causes: central sleep apnea, obstructive sleep apnea, and mixed apnea. Some sleep researchers believe that the distinctions, at least between central and obstructive apnea, are very clear; other sleep experts think the differences are blurred.

The distinction between central, obstructive, and mixed apnea is important because of their respective causes. The cause of the apnea determines treatment. Let's look at the cause of each type of sleep apnea.

Central Apnea

Pure central apnea is the least common of the three types of sleep apnea. In central apnea the cause of the breathing problem is in the brain, or central nervous system; thus the term *central apnea*. In a person with central apnea the respiratory center in the brain that controls breathing (described in Chapter 3) may simply stop working during sleep. It fails to signal the chest muscles to make breathing movements. Sleep researchers believe this may happen for a number of reasons, all related to some disorder in the breathing reflex. The disorder may be an inherited neurologic problem or a neuromuscular disorder that arises later in life, such as, post-polio syndrome, muscular dystrophy, multiple sclerosis (MS), or amyotrophic lateral sclerosis (ALS, or Lou Gehrig's disease).

A person with pure central apnea has great difficulty sleeping and breathing at the same time. As soon as he drops off to sleep, he stops breathing (Figure 4.1). When his emergency arousal response takes over, he awakens with a start and a gasp. In severe central apnea the person may get very little sleep at all. This is an extremely distressing condition that can last for many years before it is correctly diagnosed.

Another form of central apnea is sometimes seen in people who have a psychological problem called sleep onset anxiety. People with sleep onset anxiety are panicky about falling asleep. This causes them to breathe quickly and heavily, which results in a decrease in the level of carbon dioxide in their blood. When they do fall asleep, the low carbon dioxide level fails to trigger their breathing reflex for a long time. Consequently, they end up having a central apnea event and awakening to breathe.

Typically, the main complaint of a person with central apnea is that he doesn't get enough sleep. He may describe his problem as "insomnia." The reason for his complaint, of course, is his frequent awakenings during the night. However, not all people with insomnia have sleep apnea. In fact, only approximately 5 percent of insomniacs show even slight signs of sleep apnea.

Obstruction of the airway usually is not a problem in a person with pure central apnea. However, research suggests that obstructive apnea sometimes can trigger central apnea.[1] In these cases the central apnea may disappear if the airway obstruction is treated.

The long-term effects of central apnea are similar to the effects of obstructive apnea: enlargement of the heart, lung complications, and heart failure.

Drug therapy is a promising method of treating central apnea. Other treatments might involve surgery, if there are airway obstructions, and possibly the use of a nighttime ventilating device. Pacemakers for the diaphragm have also been developed and may eventually be an acceptable treatment for central apnea (see Chapter 7 for more on treatment of sleep apnea).

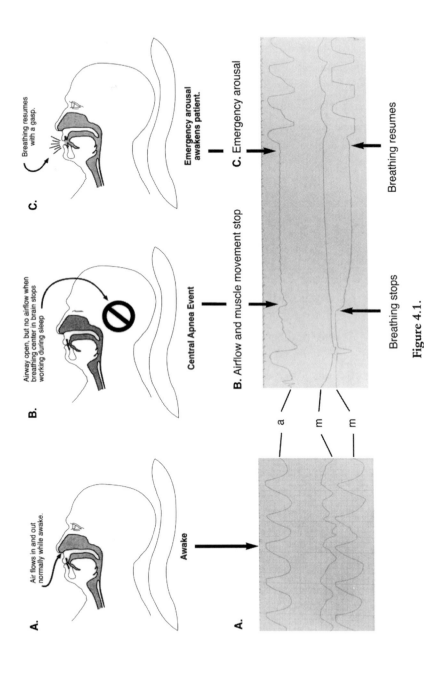

Figure 4.1.

A central apnea event. The polysomnograph tracings show the airflow in and out of the airway (a) and the movement of the breathing muscles (m). A: Normal breathing while awake. B: Breathing movements and airflow stop during sleep. C: Emergency arousal awakens the person, and he resumes breathing with a gasp.

Obstructive Sleep Apnea

In obstructive sleep apnea the upper airway is blocked during sleep by the tissue of the soft palate, throat, and/or tongue. In Chapter 3 we explained that this blockage can result from a combination of anatomic factors and irregularities in the breathing reflex.

Unlike the patient with central apnea, who simply stops breathing, the person with obstructive sleep apnea struggles to breathe against the obstructed airway (Figure 4.2). His chest moves in and out but, because of the blockage, the air cannot flow into or out of his lungs. Finally, his oxygen concentration drops, as Mr. Kennedy's did, to the point where his arousal reflex causes him to breathe. He awakens with a loud, gasping, snorting sound.

People with obstructive apnea may have one or more anatomic abnormalities associated with their upper airway: the passages in their nose and pharynx (throat) (Figure 4.3). Such abnormalities can be seen in head radiograph images of many people with obstructive sleep apnea.[2]

In the nose the abnormal structure may be a deviated nasal septum or chronic swelling of the nasal passages as a result of allergies.

In the upper pharynx obstructions may include enlarged tonsils or adenoids, an extra-long or fleshy soft palate, or a large uvula (the fleshy tab that dangles in the back of your throat.) In the lower pharynx the problem might be a large tongue, a tongue that is located unusually far back or far down, an unusually small airway opening, a short lower jaw, or a short neck.[2]

Any one of these structural features, or a combination of them, can help cause obstructive sleep apnea (Figure 4.3).

Body weight is often a factor in the development of obstructive apnea. One-half to three-fourths of patients with obstructive sleep apnea are more than 15 percent over their ideal weight.[3] Obstructive sleep apnea is common in overweight people for several reasons. First, people who are carrying extra weight usually have fatty deposits within the throat tissue, which narrow the upper airway. Second, in some heavy people the extra weight on the abdomen changes the way their

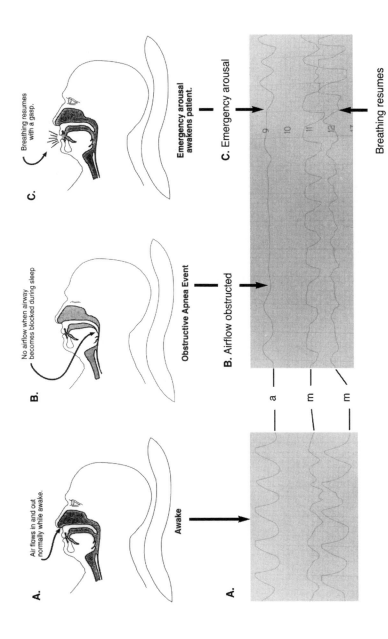

Figure 4.2

An obstructive apnea event. The polysomnograph recording shows airflow in and out of the airway (a) and the movements of the breathing muscles (m). A: Normal breathing while awake. B: The airway collapses and becomes obstructed during sleep. The breathing muscles continue to move, but no air can flow into the airway. C: Emergency arousal awakens the person, and he resumes breathing with a gasp.

stomach and chest muscles work, alters the operation of their breathing reflexes, and contributes to the development of apnea (see Chapter 8 for more on obesity and sleep apnea).

Age is also a factor in obstructive sleep apnea, as already mentioned, because the shape and muscle tone of a person's upper airway tend to change with age. Many people have no sign of obstructive sleep apnea when they are younger but develop it in their 50s or 60s (see Chapter 11 for more about age and sleep apnea).

Sex is also a factor. Obstructive sleep apnea is approximately three times more prevalent among men.

Obstructive sleep apnea is treated by attempting to remove whatever is blocking the airway. This can be accomplished by means of a breathing device, through surgery, and sometimes by both. If obesity is a factor, weight loss usually helps, if it can be maintained (see Chapter 7 for treatment of sleep apnea).

When a physician is seeking the cause, it is extremely important to very carefully determine which of these many factors are contributing to the obstructive apnea so that the most effective treatment can be chosen.

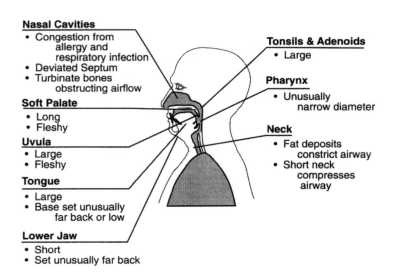

Figure 4.3
Possible sources of airway obstructions in people with obstructive apnea.

Mixed Apnea

Mixed apnea is a combination of central and obstructive apnea. Most people with sleep apnea probably have some form of mixed apnea. In fact, some sleep researchers believe that most if not all obstructive sleep apnea has a central apnea component and that some abnormality in the breathing reflex in the brain usually accompanies the development of obstructive apnea.

Others interpret the cause and effect that occur in mixed apnea a little differently. They point out that as a person gasps and recovers from an obstructive apnea event, he typically "overbreathes," which results in an unusually low level of carbon dioxide in his blood. In turn, this lower carbon dioxide level is enough to trigger a central apnea event, thereby producing mixed apnea. The more severe the obstructive apnea, the more severe the "overbreathing" is likely to be and the more obvious the central apnea component could be expected to be.

In any case, whatever the actual cause and effect in mixed apnea, the obstructive apnea is usually treated first. So you could say that, for treatment purposes, most mixed apnea is obstructive apnea. Once the breathing obstruction is treated, the central apnea will often disappear, or at least lessen to the point where it does not require treatment.

summary

- Snoring in which breathing stops is a symptom of sleep apnea.
- There are three kinds of sleep apnea:
  Central apnea, the least common type, originates in the brain;
  Obstructive sleep apnea is caused by a blockage in the airway; and
  Mixed apnea, the most common type, is a combination of central and obstructive apnea.
- The choice of treatment depends on the kind of apnea.

chapter 5

Problems and Pitfalls of Identifying Sleep Apnea

Seeking the Correct Diagnosis

The first step in treating any medical problem is, of course, the correct diagnosis. To diagnose sleep apnea correctly, two important questions need to be answered:

1. Is this condition actually sleep apnea, or is it some other disorder?

2. Is sleep apnea the only disorder present, or are other conditions present that will complicate both the sleep apnea and the treatment?

The correct diagnosis of sleep apnea can be difficult for several reasons. Sleep apnea often is confused with a number of other sleep disorders, such as narcolepsy, insomnia, restless leg syndrome, or periodic limb movement in sleep. Or the opposite can occur: other disorders (heart conditions, breathing problems, seizure disorders) can be misdiagnosed as sleep apnea. Finally, sleep apnea can be hidden or aggravated by other factors, such as certain medications (sedatives, hypnotics, and beta blockers), alcohol, depression, heart disease, obesity. For these reasons it is important for someone with suspected sleep apnea to be thoroughly tested by a sleep specialist. Incorrect or mistaken treatment can be harmful.

Difficulties in Recognizing Sleep Apnea

The diagnosis of sleep disorders is a challenge. Unlike other diseases, sleep disorders do not allow the patient to be much help to the diagnostician. The patient seldom recognizes the nature of the problem and cannot describe the most obvious symptoms because he is asleep when they occur.

Sleep specialists use polysomnography to confirm the diagnosis of sleep apnea and other sleep disorders. Polysomnography is the electronic measurement of sleep. It consists of hooking a patient up to electronic monitors, recording the patient's physiologic signals on paper during a full night's sleep, and then analyzing the recording of the electronic signals. Until these tools became available, sleep apnea went unrecognized.

Appropriately used, polysomnographic testing can distinguish between sleep disorders and other conditions and can measure their severity. Polysomnography is described in detail in the next chapter.

Even with these modern tools, however, sleep apnea can be misdiagnosed. Inappropriate sleep testing can lead to incorrect diagnosis and treatment. Tests must be done according to established standards; otherwise, the test results may be faulty. For example, testing for sleep apnea by means of daytime naps or a partial night's sleep may give a false picture. Daytime sleep is qualitatively different from nighttime sleep. Because sleep apnea often is worse during the second half of the night, when most REM sleep occurs, a partial night sleep test may miss the worst of the sleep apnea. Also, if the person sleeps poorly during a test, he may appear to have little or no apnea. Sleep apnea may actually improve with disturbed sleep and appear less severe because the person is in a lighter stage of sleep, so that the healthy, "awake" breathing center is more active than it is during a usual night's sleep.

Another reason sleep apnea has been difficult to diagnose is that most medical people are not very familiar with the condition. Only in the 1980s did doctors begin to recognize sleep apnea as a specific sleep/breathing disorder with characteristic causes and symptoms. It is still best understood by sleep specialists. Even today the average medical student receives only about 24 minutes of instruction on sleep disorders during his or her entire medical education.[1]

Unless your doctor is a recent graduate of one of the few medical schools that teach about sleep disorders, his only contact with the field may be the medical literature, which contains an occasional article about sleep disorders. Reading about sleep apnea is not the same as recognizing the symptoms in a patient. The diagnostic routines that most doctors learn in medical school never prompt them to look for the symptoms of sleep apnea.

A typical sequence of treatment begins when a physician fails to recognize the sleep apnea and attempts to treat the symptoms. Complaints of snoring, excessive daytime sleepiness (EDS), unexplained fatigue, and/or "insomnia" should be clear signals of possible sleep apnea. Instead these symptoms often are treated with drugs, such as stimulants or sleeping medications, and the underlying sleep apnea is missed or even aggravated, sometimes for many years.

Another common sequence of treatment begins when a patient first talks with a surgeon to try to solve his snoring problem. The surgeon fails to refer the patient for proper sleep testing and and does a little snoring surgery on a hunch that "you don't have sleep apnea." The snoring may improve for a while, but if the person has underlying sleep apnea, it remains undetected and untreated. The American Academy of Otolaryngology (ear, nose, and throat surgeons) has published guidelines that require patients with snoring to be properly tested before they have snoring surgery. Yet some surgeons still believe they can tell if someone has significant apnea only by talking to him!

If sleep apnea is not diagnosed or treated properly, it may become severe enough that heart and lung complications appear, as in the case of Mr. Allen (mentioned in Chapter 1). Even then, many physicians will continue to treat the symptoms without suspecting that a sleep/breathing disorder may be the cause.

The difficulties in diagnosing sleep apnea have led to an enormous amount of frustration. Sick people go from doctor to doctor, for years, tortured by sleep apnea, desperately seeking an answer. People have died, and many more have reached the brink of death, before a chance encounter (a spouse, a friend, a news article, a change of physicians) finally has brought them to a sleep center for proper testing and a clear diagnosis of sleep apnea.

Avoiding Misdiagnosis

The following are 10 rules for avoiding misdiagnosis:

1. ***Select an accredited sleep center and be evaluated by a physician who has specialized in sleep disorders.***

How can you know if the sleep center and the physician are accredited? Call the American Academy of Sleep Medicine (AASM) in Rochester, Minnesota (507-287-6006), and ask them for the nearest accredited sleep specialist or sleep center, or find a list of accredited sleep centers on their web site http://www.aasmnet.org. Or you can ask whether a particular sleep lab has been accredited by the AASM or whether a particular physician is "board certified" as a specialist in sleep disorders (see also Chapter 12).

If you live in an area without accredited sleep labs, or if you belong to an HMO that is not associated with an accredited sleep center, you may be able to find a good sleep lab that is not accredited. In that case, ask your HMO or your state medical society to refer you to a physician who has had formal training in the treatment of sleep apnea. Ask for evidence that you are being treated by a physician who is trained in sleep disorders. If it is clear that your HMO does not have access to a trained physician, consider appealing to the administration and obtain a referral to the nearest accredited sleep lab.

Accreditation is the consumer's best signpost for locating a competent sleep center. A physician earns accreditation in sleep disorders medicine by passing a rigorous two-day examination. To be sure you are being treated by someone who is a certified sleep expert, ask the following question: "Have you passed the examination for sleep specialists given by the American Board of Sleep Medicine?" If you are hesitant about asking your doctor this question directly, you can telephone his office and ask his receptionist the question. If she does not know the answer, ask her to find out and call you back.

CASE STUDY

Mr. Woods was seen at his HMO and told that he needed a sleep study. He was assured that the HMO had a "sleep lab" and that a "sleep expert" would diagnose his problem. After a night in the "sleep lab," he was told that he had central sleep apnea and was discouraged to learn that not much could be done for him.

Later Mr. Woods was studied in an accredited sleep center, where he was found to have idiopathic central nervous system (CNS) hypersomnolence, not central apnea. He also had mild sleep apnea, but it was obstructive rather than central. With medications for his idiopathic CNS hypersomnolence, he was able to return to work, and with weight loss the obstructive apnea disappeared.

CASE STUDY

Mr. Costello heard about sleep apnea and realized that he had several symptoms: heavy snoring, a weight problem, and falling asleep while driving. He discussed this with his family doctor, who gave him a continuous positive airway pressure (CPAP) machine and told him to go home and use it on a setting of "6."

Mr. Costello tried sleeping with the CPAP, but kept waking up feeling suffocated and struggling with the mask. After a week of fiddling with the CPAP setting and the mask, he gave up in frustration and returned the CPAP to the doctor's office.

A few months later Mr. Costello fell asleep at the wheel, crashed his car, and injured himself. He was referred to an accredited sleep center for a sleep study and was diagnosed with severe sleep apnea. This time the sleep center fitted him properly with a CPAP mask and custom-set the prescribed CPAP pressure for him in the sleep lab. He was surprised to find that he could sleep well with the CPAP, and within a few weeks he felt better than he had in years.

2. Be sure that your sleep study is performed at night or during your usual sleep hours.

If you are told to "stay awake all night and then come into the laboratory in the morning to have your sleep test," find another sleep center.

If you are a shift worker and are accustomed to sleeping during the day, either have your study during the day or switch back to sleeping at night *for at least three nights* before going into the lab for a sleep study at night.

CASE STUDY

Mr. Daly was told to stay up all night and then come into the sleep lab to have a sleep study. He slept poorly in the lab, and after three hours he had to end the study because he couldn't sleep any longer. He was diagnosed as having some sleep apnea and told to lose weight.

Later he was restudied properly in a nighttime sleep test at an accredited sleep center. He was found to have severe sleep apnea, particularly during the last four hours of the night, which the earlier sleep study had missed because it did not examine Mr. Daly during his usual sleep hours.

Appropriate treatment included not only weight loss but also uvulopalatopharyngoplasty (UPPP) surgery and the use of CPAP (see Chapter 7). With treatment, Mr. Daly improved remarkably and eventually was even able to discontinue CPAP.

3. *If you are sleepy while driving and working, be sure that a Multiple Sleep Latency Test (MSLT) is performed on the day following your nighttime sleep study.*

An MSLT will establish the severity of your daytime sleepiness. It also will help rule out other causes of sleepiness (e.g., other sleep disorders) and provide a baseline to refer to if fatigue and sleepiness continue after the apnea has been treated.

CASE STUDY

Ms. Jones snored badly and had been tired for years. She was sleepy when driving and couldn't stay awake during her favorite operas. She went to a "sleep lab" and was told she needed UPPP surgery.

After surgery she was pleased that she no longer snored, felt better, and was not sleepy while driving. However, she still felt tired. She was told that her trouble was related to stress and boredom.

She was restudied at an accredited sleep center and her MSLT showed that despite the surgery, she still had most of her sleep apnea. It also uncovered a second major sleep disorder that previously had been missed — narcolepsy.

4. *Be sure that you have had a recent thorough physical examination and laboratory studies, preferably with your own physician, who knows your past health problems and has all your records available.*

This will avoid duplication of tests.

CASE STUDY

Mr. Roberts was told that sleep apnea was the cause of his snoring and progressive fatigue. He had gained weight, so he was put on a weight loss program and referred to a surgeon for UPPP surgery.

He obtained a second opinion at an accredited sleep center, and physical examination found that he had low thyroid activity. Treatment eliminated his fatigue. He quickly lost the extra weight, which had also been caused by his thyroid disorder, and his apnea then disappeared.

5. **Be sure you have a thorough examination of your throat, preferably by an ear, nose, and throat specialist (also known as an ENT specialist or otolaryngologist) who is experienced with sleep apnea.**

CASE STUDY

Mr. Wilson had been told by his doctor that he probably had sleep apnea, but the doctor wouldn't refer him to a sleep center unless he lost weight. Six months later Mr. Wilson felt worse and obtained a referral from another physician.

He was found to have mild apnea, and an ENT specialist examined his throat and found a cancer narrowing his lower throat area. Mr. Wilson then realized he had been having a little trouble swallowing food, but he had not considered it to be enough of a problem to mention.

6. **If CPAP is recommended, be sure you are studied with CPAP in the sleep laboratory, so that the proper air pressure can be established to control your obstructive apnea.**

This may mean spending a second night in the laboratory. If CPAP is prescribed for you and you are simply told to "go home and try it out," find another sleep center.

CASE STUDY

Ms. Brown had heart problems, and her blood oxygen levels were checked during an evaluation for chest pain, but sleep studies were not done. Because she snored, she was told that sleep apnea was the cause of the decrease in oxygen in her blood while sleeping. She was told to go home and use CPAP.

She slept very poorly with CPAP, but she was told to keep using it because her blood oxygen was much better.

Too frightened to stop using CPAP but exhausted from not sleeping, she was studied at an accredited sleep center. She was found to have very mild apnea, but it was central apnea, not obstructive apnea, and could not be treated effectively with CPAP.

7. **If surgery, oral devices, medications, or weight loss are pre-scribed for you, be sure to have a sleep study to establish a baseline, so that it can be determined whether you are ben-efiting from the treatment, and if so how much.**
People often feel better after treatment begins and think they are "cured" when, in fact, they are only partially improved. Further treatment or careful follow-up may be necessary.

CASE STUDY

Mr. Johnson was diagnosed with severe obstructive sleep apnea. He had UPPP surgery and stopped snoring. His wife said he was cured because she "didn't notice any more apnea." Mr. Johnson felt "much better." He was told by the surgeon that a follow-up sleep study was not necessary since he obviously was cured.

Mr. Johnson's family doctor noticed that his blood pressure had not improved and convinced him to return to the sleep center. His follow-up sleep study showed that he had only improved 25 percent. The follow-ing night he was placed on CPAP. He improved more than he could have believed, and his blood pressure dropped so far that his family doctor was able to stop one of his medications.

8. *If you are diagnosed as having obstructive apnea but you
    believe that you have other reasons for feeling tired or
    drowsy or for having restless sleep, be sure to discuss them
    with your physician. It is possible that sleep apnea may not
    be the most important cause of your symptoms.*

A trial with CPAP in the sleep lab is a good way to find out how
many of your problems are caused by sleep apnea. CPAP safely eliminates any sleep apnea that you may have, and you can then be the judge
of whether you feel better or still have troublesome symptoms. If you
are in doubt about how important sleep apnea is in causing your
drowsiness, return to the laboratory for a trial with CPAP.

The opposite is also true: you may believe that you have fairly serious sleep apnea symptoms even though your sleep test may say that
your apnea is too mild for treatment. If this is the case, you may be one
of those individuals who is very sensitive to sleep disruption from
apnea. Discuss this possibility with your doctor. A trial with CPAP
would be very helpful in letting you judge how much improvement you
feel after the apnea is eliminated.

9. *If sleep studies show that your apnea is well controlled but
    you continue to be sleepy, feel fatigued, or experience sleep
    disturbances, be sure that your doctor has considered and
    ruled out other conditions that might be causing those
    symptoms.*

As many as 20 percent of patients with sleep apnea have other undiagnosed sleep disorders that may not be obvious until the sleep apnea is
diagnosed.

10. *Be sure that stress factors, depression, sleep habits, and drug
    and alcohol use have been thoroughly discussed with you.*

Unless the physician carefully questions you about these areas, they
may continue to be problems that neither you nor your doctor fully

understands! Two case studies show how unexpected factors can strongly affect the results of treatment for sleep apnea.

CASE STUDY

Mr. Williams was sent by his heart specialist to have a "sleep study." He was not seen by a sleep specialist but was told that he had significant sleep apnea, which caused his broken sleep, chronic fatigue, headaches, and drowsiness. He was sent to have UPPP surgery, and the surgeon recommended that he go to an accredited sleep center for reevaluation.

The sleep specialist discovered that Mr. Williams was very depressed and had been hiding the extent of his drug and alcohol use. Mr. Williams agreed to have drug and alcohol treatment and eventually was treated with antidepressants and counseling. His sleep disorder resolved, and a sleep study showed that he had such mild apnea that further treatment was not necessary. His alcohol use and depression had aggravated his apnea and sleep-related symptoms.

CASE STUDY

Mr. Jones went through a divorce and became depressed. He gained a lot of weight and eventually was diagnosed as having severe sleep apnea. CPAP helped somewhat, but to the dismay of both Mr. Jones and his doctor, he had no luck losing his excess weight.

Mr. Jones was still having problems with depression and finally went to see a psychiatrist. As counseling progressed and his depression lifted, he began to lose weight. He eventually had UPPP surgery, his remaining mild apnea and snoring disappeared, and he was even able to discontinue CPAP.

In Mr. Jones's case neither his sleep apnea nor his weight gain was likely to improve very much until he was treated for depression.

What Should You Do If You Think You Have Sleep Apnea?

If you think you have sleep apnea . . .

1. *First try working through your family doctor. Make an appointment and tell him or her that you think you have sleep apnea and why you think so. Ask for a referral to an accredited sleep center to be tested for sleep apnea.*

When you see your family doctor, take with you any articles or books that have helped convince you that you have sleep apnea. You might also take along a tape recording of your snoring.

If your doctor doesn't "hear" you (that is, he is not familiar with sleep apnea or does not take your diagnosis seriously) and you are still convinced you are right . . . proceed to step 2.

2. *Call the nearest accredited sleep center yourself (see the preceding section and Chapter 12). Ask for an appointment. Some sleep centers will take patients only by referral from another physician, but many centers will make appointments with patients directly.*

It is always best to work with your family doctor. If you decide to contact a sleep center directly, it still is a good idea to keep your family doctor informed. For one thing, he probably will become involved eventually because the sleep clinic will probably contact him to get your medical history. Later, as a courtesy, they probably will notify him of the treatment they recommend for you. In fact, depending on the kind of treatment, your family doctor may need to become actively involved. In addition, keeping your family doctor informed will expose him to more experience with sleep apnea, which will help other people with sleep apnea in the future.

Keep in mind that it is your health that is at stake. If your doctor seems uncooperative, you should not hesitate to get in touch with a sleep center yourself.

If the closest accredited sleep center only accepts referrals and your doctor is unwilling to refer you . . . take the next step.

3. *Ask the sleep center for one of the following:*

    a. The name of a local doctor with whom they have worked who will refer you to the sleep clinic, or

    b. The location of the closest qualified sleep center that will accept patients without a doctor's referral.

The next chapter takes you to a sleep clinic.

summary

- Sleep apnea is frequently mistaken for other conditions.

- Misdiagnosis results in incorrect treatment, sometimes with disastrous consequences.

- A specialist in sleep disorders medicine at an accredited sleep center is the physician most likely to correctly test for and diagnose sleep apnea.

- The American Academy of Sleep Medicine (AASM) can put you in touch with the nearest accredited sleep specialist or sleep center.

- The 10 rules for avoiding misdiagnosis and the "What Should You Do . . . ?" sections of this chapter will guide you toward an accurate diagnosis.

chapter 6

The Sleep Center: Testing for Sleep Apnea

The Full-Service Sleep Center

Polysomnography

Sleep specialists have developed a standard way to record and measure what is going on during a person's sleep. The procedure that is used for making these recordings is called polysomnography, which means "making multiple sleep recordings." The electronic apparatus that is used is called (not too surprisingly) a polysomnograph.

If you have ever had an electrocardiogram (ECG or EKG) or an electroencephalogram (EEG) or if you have ever seen the way a lie detector test (polygraph) is performed, you know exactly the kind of equipment that is used for polysomnography.

A polysomnograph records a person's sleep by gathering information from a set of small electrodes taped to the patient's skin. Wires lead from the electrodes to an electronic processor, which runs a row of pens. Each pen records the information that comes from one of the electrodes. The pens translate electrical brain signals into squiggly lines on a continuous, moving sheet of paper. The polysomnograph is able to run all night and record all the information from a full night's sleep on a very long, accordion-folded strip of paper. Many sleep centers also record and store these data by computer.

To study a person's sleep, each of the electrodes of the polysomnograph is attached with tape or a dab of glue to a specific location on the

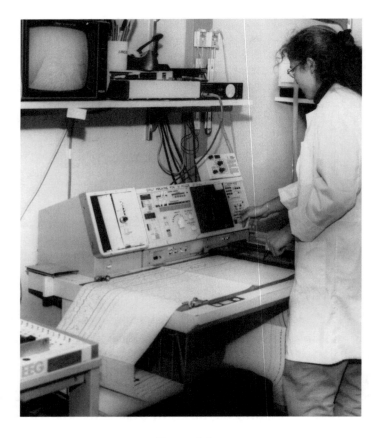

Figure 6.1
In the control room of a sleep center, a technologist monitors a patient's sleep while it is being recorded by the polysomnograph.

person's skin. The electrodes usually are placed on the following places:

- Head, as for an EEG, to record brain wave activity that distinguishes the stages of sleep and wakefulness
- Face near the outside corner of each eye, to detect eye movements
- Chin or throat, to detect jaw muscle tone
- Chest, to pick up signals of the heartbeat, as in an ECG
- Abdomen, to detect abdominal movements
- Legs, to detect abnormal leg movements

Each of these electrodes picks up information about a particular activity going on in the person's body during sleep. The recordings from each electrode can then be analyzed by comparing them with standardized "normal" recordings.

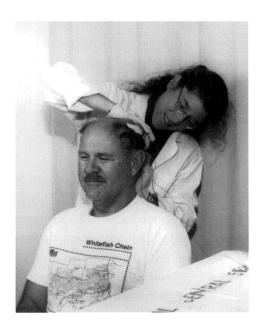

Figure 6.2
A patient being prepared for a sleep test.

When sleep apnea is being studied, several additional recordings are made to gather information about the person's breathing and to show when air is moving in and out of the airway.

- One recording wire is attached to a stretchy belt that contains a device that is fastened around the person's chest to detect expansion and contraction of the rib cage and abdomen as the muscles make breathing movements.
- Another recording device is an oximeter, which is clipped gently onto a finger or earlobe. The oximeter measures the oxygen content in the person's blood. It is able to do this without breaking the skin, so no needles are involved.
- Another device measures air moving in and out through the nose and mouth. This is done using a small detector that rests lightly on the upper lip just beneath the nose.
- In some cases, additional monitors may be used to detect other types of sleep-disordered breathing.

Once all the electrodes and other recording devices are attached to the person being studied, the wires are gathered together into a "pigtail," to keep them out of the way and avoid restricting freedom of movement. The bundle of wires plugs into a box, which leads to an adjacent room, where the bulk of the polysomnograph equipment is located.

It is important to emphasize that nothing about this recording procedure hurts! There are no needles or other pain-causing devices. The electrodes do not penetrate the skin but are simply stuck to the surface with adhesive. They will not cause an electrical shock.

The sleep study takes place in a private sleep room, which is supplied with a comfortable bed. The sleep room is very well insulated so that all outside sounds and lights are screened out, and nothing can disturb the person's sleep. The room is kept at a temperature that is comfortable for sleeping. Some sleep centers try to make the sleep rooms "homey," with carpeting, drapes, and pictures on the walls, whereas other sleep rooms look more like hospital rooms.

The Job of the Sleep Technician

Sleep technicians hook you up to the polysomnography leads, make you comfortable during the night, and monitor both your sleep and the operation of the polysomnograph equipment throughout the night. The accuracy of the results of your sleep test will depend on how carefully the technicians set you up for the test and how carefully they monitor you and the equipment. Consequently, the skill and diligence of the sleep technicians are very important.

Sleep technicians may have a wide range of training and experience, from beginners who are receiving "hands-on" training to well-trained experts who have taken courses in their field and keep up-to-date on the latest information on sleep testing and measurement techniques.

A sign of proficiency in this field is the credential of registered polysomnographic technologist (RPSGT). Sleep technicians can earn this credential by training, studying, and passing a two-day test administered by the Board of Registered Polysomnographic Technologists.

In most well-staffed sleep centers, at least the supervisor of the sleep technicians will be an RPSGT. It is important that the person in charge of the actual sleep testing have thorough understanding of the standardized procedures for setting up and carrying out a valid sleep test. Supervision by an RPSGT gives some assurance that polysomnograph equipment will be connected to the patient according to the accepted standards and that the sleep recordings will be accurate. Poorly conducted sleep tests can produce recordings that look accurate and impressive but lead to an incorrect diagnosis and may need to be repeated later on. Thus, bad sleep tests not only are a waste of your time and a waste of money for whoever is paying the bill, but also can actually result in bad medical treatment.

A Visit to a Sleep Center

Let's assume that you suspect you may have sleep apnea. Your first contact with a sleep center will probably be something like Mr. Kennedy's. His wife said, "Honey, please do something about that snoring," so he made an initial appointment with the sleep specialist at the nearest sleep center. Mrs. Kennedy was asked to come along with her husband to the initial discussion with the doctor. This is the usual procedure. One reason for both partners to be present is that your sleeping partner probably will be able to supply more information about your sleeping habits than you can. Another reason is that sleep disturbances such as sleep apnea frequently require long-term treatment, which affects both partners in some ways, so it is a good idea for both to be part of the process from the very beginning.

At the end of Mr. Kennedy's initial interview, the sleep specialist told him that he suspected sleep apnea and advised him to make an appointment for evaluation during an all-night sleep session.

Mr. Kennedy was scheduled for a date two weeks later to spend an entire night at the sleep center. He was told to plan also to spend part of the following day there for further testing. Sometimes patients spend two nights in the sleep center, but not the day in between. The testing schedule depends on the policies and procedures of the particular sleep center.

On the day of Mr. Kennedy's all-night sleep session, he was asked to arrive at the sleep center in the evening, a little before his normal bedtime, so the technician would have plenty of time to attach the electrodes and other recording devices to him. Most sleep centers ask people to avoid alcohol, narcotics, and caffeine during the day before their sleep test to eliminate any chance that these substances will interfere with sleep.

Although he knew there was nothing painful about the procedure of recording sleep, Mr. Kennedy admits to feeling some anxiety as he arrived at the sleep center. He is not alone in feeling anxious; many people are uneasy when facing an unfamiliar medical procedure.

Be sure to tell the nurses or technicians if you feel nervous whenever you are undergoing any kind of medical procedure. The medical personnel want you to be at ease. Feel free to ask questions if you are alarmed or even just curious. The technicians who prepare you for your night of sleep are so familiar with the routine that they may forget to explain the details as clearly as they should. It is okay to remind them that you are new at this and would like to understand what is going on. Everything should be clearly explained to you.

Mr. Kennedy was told that he could wear his own nightclothes as long as they fit loosely and did not interfere with the placement of the electrodes. He brought a pair of pajamas, which worked fine.

When the measuring devices had all been attached and it was approximately Mr. Kennedy's normal bedtime, the technician turned out the lights and left him to go to sleep. The technician gave him a buzzer to use in case he needed to get up during the night to use the bathroom or needed to have the technician help him with something. Then the technician would come in and unplug his wires.

Mr. Kennedy did buzz the technician once during the night. When it seemed as though a long time had passed and the technician had not appeared, Mr. Kennedy simply unclipped the oxygen sensor from his finger. The sudden change in the signal on the polysomnograph recording told the technician that Mr. Kennedy's blood oxygen had dropped to

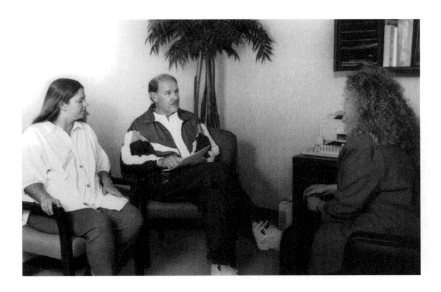

Figure 6.3
When someone suspects he has a sleep disorder, often both he and his bedmate will be asked to meet with the sleep specialist for the initial evaluation.

zero (not a good sign!). The technician arrived instantly to reattach the sensor.

You may wonder how a person can get any sleep with so many wires attached to his body. Mr. Kennedy wondered the same thing. He was sure he would never get to sleep, but the next thing he knew the technician was telling him it was morning. Despite the unusual setting, most people manage to get a fairly decent night's sleep.

The reason Mr. Kennedy was asked to stay for part of the next day was to take a multiple sleep latency test (MSLT). Sleep latency is a measure of how long it takes a person to fall asleep during the daytime. It indicates the degree of excessive daytime sleepiness (EDS) the person is experiencing. As you already know, EDS is one of the symptoms of sleep apnea.

To measure sleep latency, Mr. Kennedy was simply asked to return to his sleep room several times during the day for 20-minute rest periods. He would lie down for 20 minutes while the polysomnograph recorded whether he fell asleep and exactly how long it took him to do so.

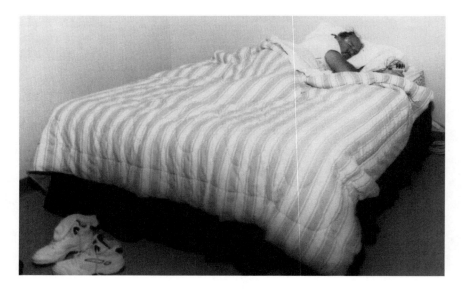

Figure 6.4
A patient asleep during a sleep test.

You will be unplugged from the recorder between MSLT naps and will be free to walk around, read, watch television, or even go to the cafeteria for lunch. Of course, you will still have all your electrodes attached and a clump of wires dangling around your neck. Some people are not bothered a bit by this. Others, like Mr. Kennedy, feel a little like Frankenstein's monster and prefer to have lunch delivered so they do not have to wander very far from the sleep center.

If you are staying in the sleep center for an MSLT, be sure to bring along something to entertain yourself: a book or magazine, crossword puzzles, needlework, or a deck of cards. If you object to wandering around in your bathrobe all day, you might bring some loose-fitting day-wear, such as a caftan or a jogging suit, which can be comfortably worn over the wires.

After all the recordings are completed, the doctor will read through the graph-paper records of your sleep night, looking for signs that tell

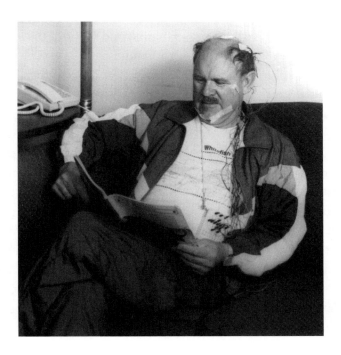

Figure 6.5
A patient killing time in the sleep center during the day between MSLTs.

him whether you have sleep apnea, and, if so, what kind and how severe it is. Another appointment will be scheduled for you to discuss the results and, if necessary, talk with you about treatment.

The "Split-Night" Sleep Study

The standard way to diagnose and treat sleep apnea requires two full nights in the sleep lab. The first night is for a diagnostic sleep study. If the sleep specialist diagnoses sleep apnea and prescribes the most common treatment, CPAP (see Chapter 7, "Treating Sleep Apnea"), the patient spends a second full night in the sleep lab so that the CPAP pressure can be custom-set for him.

In some cases, this two-night procedure is compressed into one night. This is called a "split-night" sleep study. If the patient shows signs of sleep apnea during the first half of the night, CPAP treatment is begun and the CPAP pressure is custom-set during the second half of the night.

Split-night studies have two major advantages: first, one night in the sleep lab is less expensive than two nights; and second, the sleep lab can test more patients by doing split-night studies.

However, a split-night study has several important disadvantages: it can fail to accurately show the severity of the apneas. Sleep apnea usually is worse during REM sleep, most of which occurs during the second half of the night. If a doctor is basing a diagnosis on apneas observed only during the first half of the night, he may underestimate the seriousness of a patient's sleep apnea. This is especially likely in patients who have split-night studies and are told that they have "moderate" apnea. The split-night study may miss the true severity of their apnea when sleeping in certain positions or during REM. Later, if CPAP fails to treat the patient, the insurer may refuse additional treatment, claiming that the apnea is only mild. Other problems occur when a split-night study results in diagnosing a severe patient as mild or moderate, and after CPAP fails they want to consider surgery. The surgeon may be misled by the findings of mild apnea and make ill-advised surgical recommendations. If you have a split-night study, carefully consider a full diagnostic study before having surgery.

Another possible disadvantage of a split-night study is that, even though the patient may have sleep apnea that needs treatment, the split-night may not produce enough information to convince an insurance company to pay for treatment.

Finally, there may not be enough time during the second half of the night to obtain an accurate CPAP pressure. For this reason the American Academy of Sleep Medicine does not consider split-night studies appropriate for all patients.

---

*A*t-Home Sleep Testing: Portable Monitoring

It sometimes is not necessary to spend a night in a sleep disorders center. In-home testing for sleep disorders (also called portable monitoring or ambulatory monitoring) is a new and developing field. For certain patients, and under certain conditions, the sleep specialist may suggest that the sleep study be done in the person's home.

Having a sleep study in your own home might sound to you like a better idea than spending the night in a strange place that reminds you of a hospital. Some proponents of in-home testing claim that people's sleep is more "normal" during an in-home test than in the sleep lab. However, there is no clear evidence to prove this or to prove that in-home testing is necessarily more comfortable for the patient. For some people an in-home test may have numerous drawbacks. Sleep may be disturbed by other family members, by the home surroundings, by neighborhood noises, and by other interruptions that are not present in a sleep center. On the other hand, a sleep center has a carefully regulated environment and trained technicians available in case problems arise. Furthermore, sleep specialists take into account the strangeness of the setting — which they call the "first night effect" — when they analyze the data from your sleep study in the sleep lab.

There are other important differences between an in-lab study and an in-home study. Your sleep specialist will consider these differences when deciding where you should have your sleep study.

Let's compare the two kinds of sleep studies.

TABLE 6.1

Comparison of In-Lab and In-Home Sleep Studies

	IN-LAB STUDY, ACCREDITED SLEEP CENTER	IN-HOME STUDY
Technology	Well-developed	New, still experimental
Standards exist	Yes	No
Technician training	Good	Varies from good to none
Cost	Higher	Lower
Accuracy	Good	Good to poor
Chance for errors	Low	High
Need to repeat study because of errors	Rare	Common
Paid by insurance?	Yes	Often no

When considering an in-home sleep study, you need to ask two questions:

1. What kind of in-home testing will be used?

2. For which patients is in-home testing appropriate, and are you one of them?

What kind of in-home testing is used for sleep apnea diagnosis?

In-home sleep studies vary widely in many ways. The apparatus itself can range from very simple to very complicated: from a single sensor that records the amount of oxygen in the blood to a complete "12-lead" arrangement like the polysomnography that is done in a sleep lab. How the in-home study is set up varies from one sleep lab to another. Sometimes the patient goes to the office of whoever is carrying out the study and takes the apparatus home with him. Sometimes the technician comes to the patient's home and sets up the equipment.

In 1994 the American Academy of Sleep Medicine (AASM) published its first set of recommendations on the standards and practices for portable sleep testing.[1] For diagnosing sleep apnea, the AASM's committee of sleep specialists recommended that at least four types of measurements (four "leads") are needed. Two "leads" should record breathing (breathing movements and/or airflow), and there should be one lead each for heart rate (or EKG) and oxygen in the blood. It is not good enough to measure just blood oxygen, as the simplest studies do.

Notice that with only four leads, **no information is recorded about actual sleep or sleep stages** because brain waves are not monitored. In a patient with less severe apnea, data on sleep and sleep stages often are considered necessary for diagnosing sleep apnea. This is why a person with less serious sleep apnea symptoms may need to go to a sleep lab for a complete, polysomnographic sleep study, while, paradoxically, a patient with more severe symptoms may be diagnosed by a simpler sleep study in his own home.

Whether the sleep study is "attended" or "unattended" is another issue. Some in-home studies are "attended," which means either that a technician remains in the home to monitor the study or that the patient is monitored remotely by the sleep lab, so that if something goes wrong, the sleep lab technician knows immediately and can call the patient's home and solve the problem. Many things can go wrong during a sleep study. Equipment has been known to fail during the night, and it is not unusual for electrodes to come loose from the patient's skin when he moves around during sleep. If no technician is present to fix the problem, the results of the sleep study may be worthless. Studies that are "unattended" may need to be repeated if something goes wrong during the night. Repeating sleep studies is expensive, which explains why some insurance providers are reluctant to pay for in-home sleep studies. The AASM guidelines recommend that all sleep studies be attended studies.[2]

Another issue with in-home sleep testing is the training and skill of the staff carrying out the test. A test set up by a poorly trained technician or analyzed by an unqualified person may generate misleading results. The AASM standards specify that only a licensed physician may order an in-home sleep test, and that the individuals who set up and evaluate the test should be certified or eligible for certification. However, at present the consumer has no assurances about the training or qualifications of technicians conducting in-home studies.

For which patients is in-home testing appropriate?

The 1994 recommendations by the AASM suggest that in-home testing may be appropriate in the following cases:

1. For patients who have obvious, severe symptoms and seem very likely to have sleep apnea (habitual snoring, excessive daytime sleepiness, obesity, and observed apneas), an in-home study can be used basically to confirm the diagnosis of sleep apnea in order to start treatment as soon as possible.

2. An in-home or portable study may be used for patients who cannot get to a sleep lab because they either are too ill to be moved or live too far away from a sleep disorders center.

3. For a follow-up sleep study, after a patient has been diagnosed and treated for a while, an in-home test can be used to see whether the treatment has been effective.

If an in-home sleep study is suggested to you, ask how many measurements will be recorded. Will there be at least four "leads," as recommended by the AASM? Do not accept assurances lightly.

Unless you have very obvious sleep apnea (habitual snoring, excessive daytime sleepiness, obesity, and observed apneas) that mainly just needs to be confirmed, you should make sure that the sleep study will actually monitor your *sleep*. This means that sensors should be attached to your head to monitor brain waves (EEG), eye movements (EOG), and chin movements (EMG) as well as heart rate, breathing or airflow, oxygen saturation, and body movements.

In-home testing has some strong advocates. Among these are some small sleep labs that are not equipped to test large numbers of patients. The ability to test patients at home is an advantage for such labs.

Homecare providers and medical equipment manufacturers are also expanding into the business of in-home testing. Generally, they supply the equipment, send a technician to the patient's home to set up the test, and send the results to a physician for analysis. The AASM recommends against any arrangement in which the company conducting the test stands to profit from the results by selling the patient a CPAP unit or homecare services. The possibility for conflict of interest here is obvious.

Unless and until professional standards such as those recommended by the AASM are agreed upon and followed, in-home testing can be expected to vary widely in its accuracy and cost-effectiveness.

---

*D*etermining the Severity of Sleep Apnea

When is a person's sleep apnea severe enough to cause concern? Sleep specialists define "clinical" sleep apnea (sleep apnea that needs medical attention) in the following terms:

- An *apnea event* is when breathing stops for more than 10 seconds.
- A *hypopnea event* is a partial apnea in which airflow in and out of the lungs is reduced for 10 seconds or more.
- A person is considered to have "clinical" sleep apnea if he has more than five apnea or hypopnea events per hour.

This definition determines whether the person has sleep apnea, but it tells only part of the story.

The next question is "How severe is the sleep apnea?" How sick is this person? The sleep specialist needs to answer this question to decide on the appropriate treatment.

Sleep specialists use several "yardsticks" to determine the severity of a person's sleep apnea. The simplest measure, now somewhat outdated, is called the *apnea index*. This is just the number of apnea events per hour of sleep: a person who has 30 apnea events per hour of sleep would have an apnea index of 30.

Another measurement is the total number of apnea events during an entire night. As an example, 250 apneas in an eight-hour night would not be unusual for a person with moderately serious sleep apnea.

A more accurate measure than the apnea index is the *Apnea-plus-Hypopnea Index (AHI),* also called the *Respiratory Disturbance Index (RDI).* The AHI (or RDI) expresses the total number of apneas plus hypopneas. The combined totals are a better measure of the severity of sleep apnea because apneas and hypopneas are equally important in causing the symptoms of sleep apnea.

Even the RDI may not give the full picture of sleep apnea severity. Another important indicator is oxygen saturation — the amount of oxygen present in the blood. Some people, despite a fairly small number of apnea events, may still be quite sick because of a very low oxygen saturation level. So the measurement of oxygen saturation is an important part of the total sleep apnea picture. Oxygen saturation is measured as a percentage. Normal is about 95 percent, and it decreases slightly as we get older. In people with sleep apnea, a blood oxygen content of approximately 80 percent during sleep is fairly common. Levels below 70 percent are considered critically low because of the high probability of irregular heart rhythm at lower blood oxygen levels.

Recently another indicator has been proposed, the *respiratory-arousal index (RAI).* This is the total number of arousals per hour of sleep from apneas, hypopneas, and all other sleep-disordered breathing events combined.

A further aspect of the severity of sleep apnea and the need for treatment is the question of daytime sleepiness: Is sleepiness interfering with the person's life? Some people are more sensitive to sleepiness than others, and alertness is more critical for some than for others (e.g., an airplane pilot or a school bus driver). The results of the multiple sleep latency test (MSLT), described earlier, give a good measurement of a person's tendency to fall asleep during the day.

---

*W*ho Needs Treatment?

After your sleep test, in a follow-up visit or phone call, your sleep specialist will review your sleep test results with you: RDI, oxygen saturation record, MSLT. These data and consideration of your overall health will help him decide whether your sleep apnea is serious enough to need treatment.

People usually need immediate treatment if their excessive drowsiness interferes with such daily activities as driving, if it creates job hazards, if they have heart failure related to sleep apnea, or if they have very low oxygen saturation during the night. People who constantly feel tired or who have worsening high blood pressure, heart arrhythmias related to sleep apnea, badly disrupted sleep, or an RDI of more than 20 also usually need treatment.

If a person's symptoms are less severe or the results of the sleep study show mild sleep apnea, the sleep specialist needs to carefully consider the whole picture before deciding whether to recommend treatment

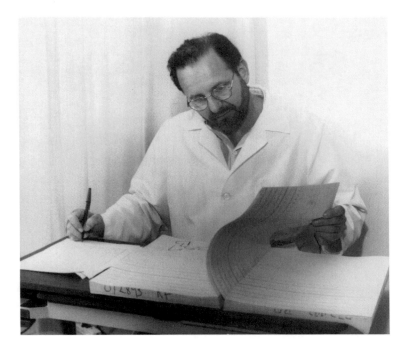

Figure 6.6
A trained sleep center staff member studies and "scores" the results of a polysomnograph test. The score indicates the kind of sleep disorder and its severity. The paper on this table is the result of one patient's sleep test.

and, if so, how aggressive the treatment should be. See Chapter 7 for treatment of sleep apnea.

summary

- Sleep testing involves sleeping for a night at a sleep center while a device called a polysomnograph electronically records your sleep.
- You may also be asked to spend part of the next day at the sleep center for a Multiple Sleep Latency Test (MSLT).
- From the results of these tests, the sleep specialist will: Decide whether you have sleep apnea; and, if so, Determine how severe it is; and Rule out other disorders that might accompany the sleep apnea.

chapter 7

Treating Sleep Apnea

C A S E   S T U D Y

Mr. Kennedy had a complete sleep test at an accredited sleep center. The test results showed that he had more than 250 apnea events during the night while his sleep was being recorded. His sleep specialist told him that he had moderately severe obstructive sleep apnea with a minor central apnea component, as well as cardiac arrhythmia. The specialist recommended that he undergo treatment.

At this point, Mr. Kennedy had answers to the first two questions on the pathway to successful treatment of sleep apnea:

1. Is his condition actually sleep apnea, and does he have any other conditions that will have a bearing on successful treatment?

2. What kind of sleep apnea is it (central, obstructive, or mixed), and how severe is it? (The answer to this question is important because it determines the kind of treatment.)

Finally comes the third and crucial question:

3. What is the best treatment for Mr. Kennedy's type of sleep apnea?

Choosing the Best Treatment

The best treatment for anyone is the most conservative treatment that will succeed in his particular situation. What is the most conservative treatment that will work for you? After a diagnosis has been made, this is a complex and individual question that should be explored carefully by you, your sleep specialist, and perhaps your family doctor. The treatment should be chosen on the basis of the kind of apnea, how severe it is, and your overall health. Your sleep specialist can describe the various treatments that may be effective for you and can tell you which ones are the most conservative.

What do we mean by *most conservative?* This means the treatment that carries the lowest risk for *you.*

Keep in mind that different doctors may have different treatment recommendations. Every doctor has conscious and unconscious biases in favor of certain forms of treatment. This is a natural result of his or her training, specialization, and personal experience. For example, a surgeon is more likely than an internist to believe that surgery is the best option; an internist might lean toward nonsurgical treatment.

Your job is to take these possible biases into account as you and your doctors weigh the risks and benefits and choose the most appropriate treatment for you.

Some treatment options involve surgery. It is always wise to get a second opinion from a different physician before deciding on surgery.

The most conservative treatments for sleep apnea do not involve surgery. They may involve some inconvenience or perseverance, but they do not expose the patient to the risks of pain and possible complications or death that are inherent in any surgical procedure.

After the nonsurgical options, the next most conservative treatments are the simplest surgical procedures. A surgical procedure can be considered "simple" if it meets most or all of the following criteria:

- It is a routine procedure that has been carried out for many years rather than a new or experimental type of surgery.
- It does not involve cutting major blood vessels or nerves, dealing with major organs, or entering a body cavity.
- It normally has no serious postoperative complications.
- It can be performed by a surgeon who is experienced with this particular surgical procedure.
- It can be done on an outpatient basis or involves, at most, a minimal (one- or two-day) hospital stay.

Surgery has many potential pitfalls: pain, excessive loss of blood, reactions to medications, nerve or muscle damage, infection, wound breakdown, and other complications.[1,2]

One of the biggest risks from surgery is general anesthesia.[1] This is particularly true for a person with sleep apnea. Anesthetics depress the breathing reflexes, and a person with sleep apnea already has some degree of respiratory difficulty. Anyone with sleep apnea who is having surgery should warn his surgeon in advance that he has sleep apnea. Better yet, he could ask his sleep specialist to consult with the surgeon. The surgeon and the anesthesiologist should both be aware that this person's breathing will need to be monitored very carefully during and immediately after surgery.

So even "simple" surgery should be considered very carefully. Surgery may be the only option that makes sense for a person who is very sick as a result of sleep apnea — it may be necessary to save his life. For other people who are not in immediate danger from the severe long-term effects of apnea or who may simply want to "stop snoring," the potential risks involved in some of the surgical procedures may outweigh the possible benefits.

It is extremely important to realize that the surgical procedures for sleep apnea are not equally effective for all people. For example, the earliest surgical procedure that was used for sleep apnea and is still being used today is uvulopalatopharyngoplasty (UPPP) (described later). As a treatment for sleep apnea, UPPP has about a 50 percent failure rate, and after five years the success rate may fall to as low as 25 percent. This means that 50 percent of the people who undergo this surgery still have a significant problem with sleep apnea immediately after surgery, and the percentage of people with problems will increase with time.

Surgery for reconstructing the lower jaw (mandibular advancement and its variations) also has a fairly high nonsuccess rate.

There are several reasons for the failure of surgery to correct sleep apnea. One is simply inappropriate choice of treatment. There are some patients for whom it can be predicted in advance that UPPP is not likely to cure their apnea. Yet some of these patients choose to have surgery anyway. Quite often, after a person is told he has sleep apnea, he is not ready to think of himself as having a long-term health condition. He may seize upon surgery as a hopeful "quick fix." Or the person may be referred directly to a surgeon by a family doctor who is unfamiliar with or biased against nonsurgical treatments for sleep apnea. Poor surgical candidates usually find that their sleep apnea returns after surgery and that they still need long-term treatment.

Another reason for the low success rate of surgery is the newness of treating sleep apnea with surgery. There still are not enough data to be able to predict accurately which people will be cured by a particular reconstructive procedure.

Before you choose surgery for the treatment of sleep apnea, ask your sleep specialist about the chances of success for you, and listen carefully to his answer.

To summarize, it makes sense to be sure you are an excellent candidate for the particular kind of surgery you are considering before you take the risk of having it. A second opinion from a qualified sleep specialist who will not be performing the surgery is strongly advised.

One final point on choosing a conservative treatment: If you are considering being treated at a medical school, you might keep in mind that medical schools may lean toward more aggressive, more experimental, less conservative treatment options. Although this is fine from the point of view of advancing medical science, ask yourself whether you want to risk being part of that process.

Does Insurance Pay for Sleep Apnea Treatment?

You will want to contact your insurance provider when you begin to consider treatment for sleep apnea. Ask them which treatments they will pay for and exactly what that coverage includes. Most insurance providers now pay for the most common treatments for sleep apnea if the treatment is prescribed by a sleep specialist. However, some surgical procedures may not be covered.

Who Treats Sleep Apnea?

Where your treatment will be carried out will depend both on your sleep center and on the treatment you will have. Some sleep centers provide both testing and treatment of sleep apnea, some do only sleep testing, and some fall in between these two extremes, doing some types of treatment in-house but referring patients elsewhere for others.

In any case, you can expect the sleep specialist and his staff to work with you and your family to plan your treatment and to recommend a treatment specialist. Your family doctor may be brought into the process at this stage.

Your sleep doctor may begin by suggesting a number of treatments that you can carry out on your own (stop smoking, lose weight, and so on). To help you with these, the sleep center may refer you to a nutritional counselor, a smokers' support group, or other such organized programs.

If surgery is an option for you and your sleep center does not perform surgery, the center will probably suggest or recommend surgeons and other specialists with whom its staff members work frequently, and these physicians will be brought into the picture to help plan your treatment.

If your sleep center has surgeons and other specialists on the staff who can treat you there, you may still want to talk with an outside physician, preferably one with some familiarity with sleep disorders, for a second opinion before you agree to surgery.

If your treatment involves medications, the sleep center may prefer to start you on the medication and then have your family physician take over the follow-up care and monitor your progress.

The most common treatment involves the use of a breathing device. The device may be supplied through the sleep center, or the center may arrange for a homecare or medical equipment company to supply the equipment.

How you receive your treatment will depend on the particular sleep center, the size of its staff, and the emphasis of its program (see Chapters 13 through 15 for more information on how to obtain the health care services you need).

---

*T*he First Step in Treatment: Eliminate the Obvious

The first step in treating sleep apnea is to eliminate anything that is aggravating your problem. This may improve your symptoms enough that you can avoid more complicated forms of treatment. The following can all increase symptoms:

- Alcohol, especially in the evening (even a single glass of wine with dinner), can increase the number of apnea events and decrease the level of oxygen in the blood during the night. A person with sleep apnea should avoid alcohol in the evening.

- Smoking decreases the amount of oxygen in the blood. It also causes swelling of the lining of the airway, which contributes to obstructive apnea. People with sleep apnea would be wise to stop smoking.

- Allergies and respiratory infections also cause swelling and obstruction of the airway. Treatment of allergies and upper airway infections can diminish the symptoms of obstructive sleep apnea.

- Evening medications, such as tranquilizers and short-acting beta blockers, sometimes can worsen sleep apnea. The sleep specialist may want to consult the physician who prescribed the medication to see whether a change in prescription or in medication schedule can help eliminate sleep apnea symptoms (see Appendix for list of medications that affect sleep).

- Obesity contributes greatly to obstructive sleep apnea, and weight loss can help or even eliminate sleep apnea. Weight loss is discussed in detail later in the section on treating obstructive sleep apnea and in Chapter 8.

- Shift work. Anything that interferes with the amount and quality of sleep (as shift work does) can worsen sleep apnea symptoms. Ask your sleep specialist for information on how to improve your sleep while on shift work. You may even want to consider changing to a job that does not require rotating shifts.

Some of these aggravating factors involve lifestyles and habits that are difficult to change or to give up. Often people have the best results if they are enrolled in an organized program to help them eliminate the habit. If you find yourself trying to deal with a stubborn problem such as losing weight or stopping smoking, ask your sleep center to recommend a program that has been helpful for other people.

*T*reatments for Central Apnea

Drugs

Drugs that stimulate the breathing reflexes are presently the most common treatments for central apnea. Unfortunately, most of the drugs have drawbacks that make them less than ideal. Some are not very effective; some work for a while, but the person may develop a tolerance to the drug; and some have undesirable side effects. Consequently, the drugs available today for treating central apnea should be considered temporary measures, and we must hope that research in this field will soon offer more acceptable alternatives.

Acetazolamide is the drug that has received the most attention. It makes the blood more acidic, which tends to stimulate the breathing reflex. Experiments have shown that acetazolamide can decrease the number of apnea events and result in a modest decrease in daytime sleepiness.[3] Other studies are less enthusiastic,[4] and there are reports of this drug leading to the development of obstructive apnea.[5] More research is needed, but at the present time acetazolamide is the most promising drug for the treatment of central apnea.

Another drug that has provided some improvement in central apnea is *clomipramine,* which is an antidepressant. It has been used on only a few patients and has resulted in improved sleep and respiration and fewer apnea events. However, some patients developed a tolerance to the drug after 6 to 12 months, after which it was no longer effective. In addition, clomipramine has some undesirable side effects, one of which is impotence.[6,7]

A third drug that has been tried experimentally on central apnea with some encouraging results is *doxapram,*[6] which is a respiratory stimulant that normally is used only for the short term (one or two hours at a time) to stimulate the breathing of patients who are recovering from anesthesia. It has never been recommended for long-term use, and it has some serious side effects, including hyperactivity, irregular heart rhythms, increased blood pressure, nausea and diarrhea, and urinary retention. It should not be used in people with heart disease, high blood pressure, or perhaps heart rhythm irregularities. These categories include many people who have serious complications from sleep apnea. It remains to be seen how useful this drug will be.

Other drugs that have been tried, with very little improvement in the central apnea, are *aminophylline* and *theophylline,* both of which are bronchodilators normally used to treat asthma and emphysema; *almitrine,* a breathing stimulant; *naloxone,* a drug that has been used to counteract the depression of the breathing reflexes that results from morphine, codeine, and so on; *medroxyprogesterone,* a hormone similar to the female hormone progesterone, which is known to stimulate respiration; and *tryptophan,* an amino acid that reportedly acts as an antidepressant. None of these medications has had dramatic effects on central apnea. All of them except tryptophan can have serious undesirable side effects.[6,12]

Oxygen has also been tried, with mixed results.[13] It is useful in more severe cases in conjunction with CPAP and/or bi-level PAP (CPAP is described in a subsequent section).

With so many drugs in existence and new ones being developed each year, one hopes that drugs will soon be found that provide a specific treatment for people with central apnea without serious side effects. Much more vigorous research in this field is needed.

Breathing Devices

DIAPHRAGMATIC PACEMAKER

A *diaphragmatic pacemaker* works very much like a heart pacemaker. It uses tiny, rhythmic pulses of electric current to stimulate rhythmic muscle contractions. Diaphragmatic pacemakers were first developed to treat polio patients whose breathing reflexes were damaged. However, the devices were never used much for this purpose because "iron lungs" were developed and the availability of the polio vaccine soon eliminated the need.

Since then some work has been done using diaphragmatic pacemakers in patients with spinal cord injuries whose breathing reflexes have been interrupted, and in infants born with faulty breathing reflexes. A few diaphragmatic pacemakers have been tried on adult patients with central sleep apnea.

In theory, this seems like an ideal solution. Central apnea is essentially the absence of the nerve signal that goes to the diaphragm during sleep to tell it to breathe. A pacemaker used during sleep should be able to supply that signal. However, this technology has not advanced very rapidly, and the diaphragmatic pacemaker has not yet become widely available, probably partly because until recently the demand was not there. Demand may increase with better recognition of central sleep apnea.

Implanting the pacemaker requires delicate surgery to place a pair of tiny electrodes next to the phrenic nerves (the nerves that control the diaphragm). This is done either in the neck, using a local anesthetic, or in the chest cavity, under anesthesia. Usually both nerves, one on each side of the body, are used rather than just one, which would only stimulate one side of the diaphragm. A small receiver also is placed underneath the skin during surgery.[14,15] To use the pacemaker, a radio frequency generator is placed against the skin over the implanted receiver, and radio frequency pulses stimulate the phrenic nerve.

Some problems and risks are involved in using a diaphragmatic pacemaker in a person with sleep apnea. One drawback is that it can cause obstructive apnea to emerge, which raises a new set of issues.[16] The most serious risk is the possibility of damaging the phrenic nerve, either during surgery or at some later time. Of course, loss of both phrenic nerves would leave the person with a paralyzed diaphragm and unable to breathe well on his own. For this reason the operation must be done with meticulous care to avoid the slightest damage to the nerves.

If you are considering this type of surgery, you would be wise to go to whatever lengths are necessary to locate a medical center that has an extensive history of installing and using diaphragmatic pacemakers and to find the surgeon who is most experienced with the procedure.

At present a diaphragmatic pacemaker probably is not a practical treatment option for most people with central apnea, although it may be considered for some patients. As research is done and experience is gained, these devices may become a more attractive method of treatment.

MECHANICAL VENTILATORS

Several forms of mechanical breathing systems can be used to assist breathing during sleep by people with central apnea. These devices operate either by "positive pressure" (forcing air into the lungs in a rhythmic, breathing-like pattern) or by "negative pressure" (more or less mimicking the actions of the breathing muscles).

Positive-pressure ventilators operate by rhythmically pushing air into the airway through a tube. The air tube usually enters the body by way of a tracheostomy, a direct opening in the throat (described later). In emergencies or in very sick people, however, the tube may be inserted through the nose or mouth, or the person may be ventilated with a face mask or nasal mask.

A positive-pressure ventilator is less cumbersome than a negative-pressure ventilator, and its use is becoming more common as better ventilators and face masks become available.

A negative-pressure ventilator works differently. The best-known example of a negative-pressure ventilator probably is the "iron lung," which was developed in the 1930s to "breathe" for polio victims who had lost their breathing reflexes. An iron lung works by rhythmically lowering the air pressure in a chamber surrounding the person's body. When the pressure around the body drops, the lungs expand and air flows into them. Your diaphragm normally operates in exactly this way — by contracting downward it lowers the pressure inside your rigid chest cavity and allows your lungs to expand and fill with air.

A number of miniaturized versions of the iron lung have been developed that surround only the chest. One such system is called a cuirass, named for the rigid piece of armor that was worn over the upper body by medieval knights. The ventilator cuirass fits closely over the chest of the person lying in bed. The cuirass is connected to an air pump, which rhythmically lowers the pressure between the cuirass and the chest, enabling air to enter the lungs. The seal between the shield and the body must be very good for the cuirass to work effectively. Some people have difficulty getting a good fit.

Mechanical ventilators have had their problems. The rhythm can be tricky to adjust; it must be regulated to breathe at the proper rate for the person using it. A mechanical system that completely controls breathing is uncomfortable for people who are somewhat able to breathe on their own and need only occasional assistance. The newest generation of ventilators minimizes this discomfort by allowing the person to breathe on his own as much as he can and to assist breathing only if he stops.

Although cumbersome, these breathing systems can be effective for many people who have central apnea and are unable to sleep and breathe at the same time.

CONTINUOUS POSITIVE AIRWAY PRESSURE

Continuous positive airway pressure (CPAP) is a breathing system that has been used successfully to treat obstructive sleep apnea. It was devised in 1981 by Sullivan and his group at the University of Sydney Medical School in Australia.[17]

A few patients with central apnea have been tried on CPAP with some success.[18] Some patients who appear to have central sleep apnea may improve on nasal bi-pressure therapy (such as BiPAP®). Others will have little if any improvement. Treatment of central apnea is still being investigated. (For more information about CPAP and BiPAP®, see the later section on treating obstructive sleep apnea.)

The choice of treatment for central apnea should be made only after a thorough consultation with your sleep specialist.

---

*T*reatments for Obstructive and Mixed Apneas

Obstructive and mixed apnea are easier to treat than central apnea. The current methods of treating obstructive sleep apnea are (from most conservative to least conservative) change of sleeping position, weight loss, breathing devices, oral devices, drugs, and surgery.

Mixed apnea generally is treated by first treating the obstructive apnea component. Once the obstructive apnea is under control, the central apnea almost always ceases to be a problem.

Change of Sleep Position

People with obstructive sleep apnea generally have more severe apnea events when sleeping on their back; a few people have breathing difficulties *only* while lying on their back. A change in sleep position may eliminate the problem for these few people. However, there is no good evidence that this technique produces reliable results each night.

Even if sleep testing shows fewer breath-holds in a particular position, airflow may still be poor enough to cause sleep disruption. If you feel better rested on CPAP than you do simply sleeping on your side without CPAP, you have good evidence that you need more than positional treatment.

Some people's apnea is so severe that even brief periods of apnea are life-threatening, and position training is not helpful.

Position change is helpful primarily to people who

1. Have obstructive apnea that has been shown during a sleep study to occur only while lying on their back; and

2. Can reliably sleep on their side.

Learning to avoid a particular sleep position is a matter of conditioning. Several sleep position monitors and alarms have been developed that alert the sleeper when he rolls onto his back and train him to choose a different sleep position. Two simple methods are sewing a small ball into the back of the pajamas or wearing to bed a small rucksack containing a bulky object that will make you lie on your side. People usually need a couple of weeks of practice before a new sleep position becomes a habit and may need to "retrain" themselves periodically.

Weight Loss

WHO CAN BE HELPED BY WEIGHT LOSS?

Weight loss can be effective for people with the Pickwickian syndrome (see Chapter 8) and many other overweight heavy snorers:

1. Whose apnea is associated primarily with their weight gain rather than with an anatomic obstruction of the airway (such as stuffy nose, large tonsils); and

2. Whose life is not in immediate danger from the effects of sleep apnea, such as sleepiness or heart disease.[19-21]

The people who are most likely to be successful at weight loss are overweight apnea sufferers who are highly motivated to improve their health and lifestyle.

WHY DOES WEIGHT LOSS WORK?

When it is effective, weight loss works for two reasons. It relieves the abnormal loading on the abdomen that interferes, in some cases, with breathing reflexes; and it reduces the fatty deposits in the throat tissue that contribute to the development of obstructive apnea. However, weight loss is only effective if:

1. Sufficient weight is lost; and

2. The weight can be kept off permanently.

Insufficient weight loss and weight regained are the two main reasons for failure of this treatment when it does fail. In fact, there may be a kind of weight "threshold," above which extra weight causes apnea symptoms and below which the symptoms are relieved.[19] According to this theory, you need to reduce your weight far enough to fall below that threshold before you can expect to see significant improvement in your apnea symptoms.

Losing weight and keeping it off may be difficult or impossible for some people as long as their sleep apnea is untreated. Their fatigue, sleepiness, low energy, and reduced vigor may prevent them from being

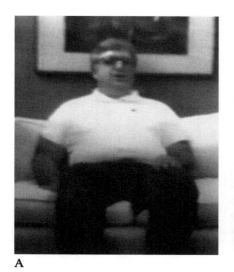
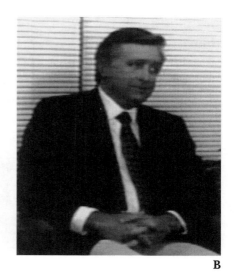

A   B

Figure 7.1
A successful weight loss patient, (A) before treatment for sleep apnea, and (B) five years later.

physically active enough to burn calories, build muscle, and successfully lose weight. In these cases the combination of CPAP (discussed later) and weight loss can have dramatic results (Figure 7.1). (For more on obesity, sleep apnea, and weight loss, see Chapter 8.)

Weight loss surgery is a radical way to lose weight. It is not a conservative treatment and is discussed later in the section on surgery.

CPAP and Similar Breathing Devices

Breathing devices that treat obstructive apnea do so by using air pressure as a "splint" to hold the upper airway open and keep it from collapsing during sleep. Some sleep experts believe that, in addition, the higher than normal air pressure delivered by these devices may stimulate the person's breathing reflexes. However, the primary role of air pressure devices is to act as an airway splint.

The most commonly used version of this system is called CPAP (pronounced "SEE-pap"). As mentioned previously, CPAP was developed as a treatment for sleep apnea by Sullivan and his research group in

Australia in 1981.[17] It was first used to treat sleep apnea patients in the United States in 1984.

CPAP is extremely effective. In fact, it is the most effective nonsurgical treatment for obstructive sleep apnea. For that reason, CPAP has become the treatment of choice at most sleep centers.

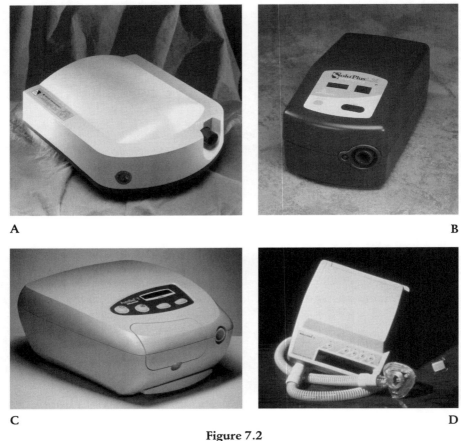

A   B

C   D

Figure 7.2
Examples of CPAP units.
(A) GoodKnight™ 314, by Mallinckrodt Nellcor Puritan Bennett. Size 4″ × 9″ × 10″, 5.3 lbs.
(B) Solo™ Plus, by Respironics. Size 10″ × 5.5″ × 4.25″, less than 5 lbs. Similar in appearance are the Aria® and the Virtuoso® smart CPAP (both 3.5 lbs).
(C) AutoSet® T, by ResMed, a smart CPAP. Size 5.7″ × 10.2″ × 12.4″, 7.7 lbs.
(D) SULLIVAN® V, by ResMed. Size 4.1″ × 9.5″ × 11″, 4.5 lbs.

The standard CPAP system consists of a small, soft, rubbery mask that is worn over the nose (not the mouth) at night. The mask is connected by flexible tubing to an air pump, which provides continuous air pressure through the tubing and into the nose (Figures 7.2 and 7.3). As soon as the CPAP wearer begins to inhale, the air pressure stabilizes his

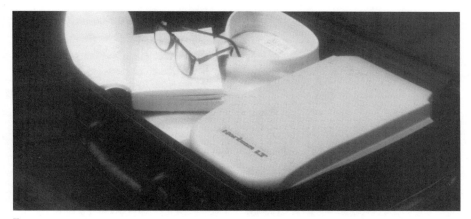

E

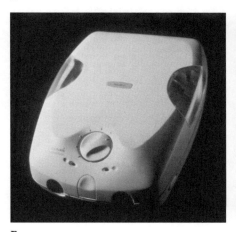

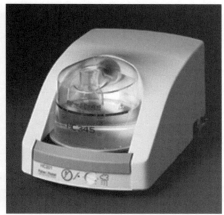

F   G

Figure 7.2 *(cont.)*

(E) Horizon® LT, by DeVilbiss®. Size 4″ × 7.7″ × 10.3″, 3.6 lbs.

(F) SULLIVAN® HumidAire™ heated humidifier by ResMed, 5.2 lbs.

(G) Fisher & Paykel Humidified CPAP System, the first to combine both functions in one unit.

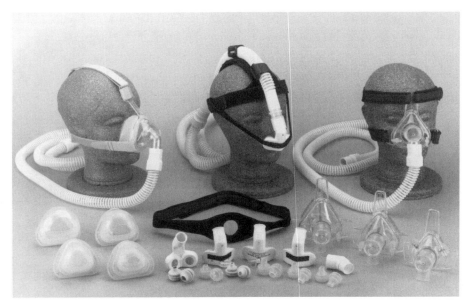

A

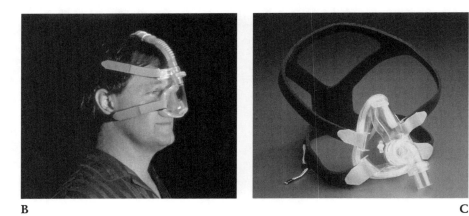

B   C

Figure 7.3

Examples of CPAP masks.

(A) Mallinckrodt Nellcor Puritan-Bennett offers a variety of masks. Left: the SoftFit™ nasal mask system, silicone cushion. The Companion® is similar, with vinyl cushion. Center: the ADAM system, the nasal pillows that fit into the nostrils are available in 6 sizes. Right: SULLIVAN® Nasal Bubble Mask®, cushion available in several series and sizes.

(B) Mirage™ nasal mask by ResMed. Available in 2 sizes.

(C) Mirage™ full face mask by ResMed.

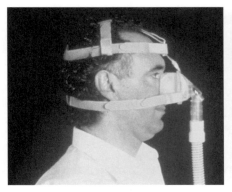

D

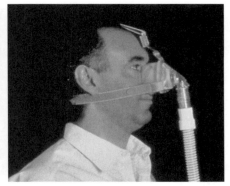

E

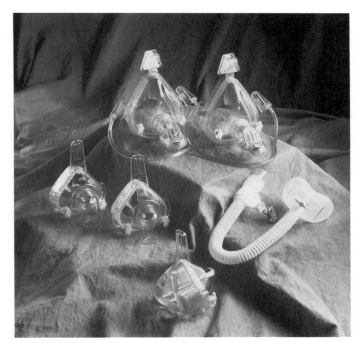

F

Figure 7.3 *(cont.)*

(D) and (E) Some ResMed headgear options for their SULLIVAN® Bubble masks.

(F) Respironics masks, clockwise from top: two full-face masks cover nose and mouth (available in 4 sizes); the Monarch® Mini Mask, the Ultra version has a swivel where the tubing attaches; the GoldSeal™ gel cushion mask (available in 7 sizes); two Contour Nasal Masks (available in 8 sizes).

soft palate and tongue and prevents his airway from collapsing. A pressure regulator is custom-set for him during a night in the sleep lab so that the CPAP delivers exactly enough air pressure to prevent his apnea events, but no more than necessary.

CPAP pressure is measured in centimeters of water (cm H_2O), in much the same way that barometric pressure is measured in millimeters of mercury (mm Hg). Typical CPAP pressure settings range from 5 to 20 cm H_2O.

In some severe cases of obstructive sleep apnea, oxygen may be prescribed in conjunction with CPAP or bi-level PAP.

Bi-level PAP (called BiPAP® by one manufacturer) is a refinement of CPAP. This system allows the air pressure to be set at two different levels. The pressure as the person inhales can be set higher to eliminate snoring, and the pressure during exhaling can be set lower, making it easier to exhale.

A new, developing, and experimental type of CPAP is often referred to as a "smart-PAP." This machine attempts to change pressure in response to the user's needs. The device senses the user's breathing patterns and adjusts pressure to accommodate changes in breathing that occur throughout the night. There are several manufacturers of smart-PAPs, and each one uses different breathing signals to regulate their machines. Some designs are more comfortable for the user than others, and some are more appropriate for certain types of users.

These dual- and variable-pressure systems are now the prescribed treatment of choice for certain severe sleep apnea patients. However, at the time of this writing, the cost of such systems is still two or more times that of a standard CPAP, and there is little evidence of improved results. For many people with sleep apnea, the advantages probably would not justify the extra cost, nor would most insurance or health plans pay for the extra "bells and whistles" of a bi-level or smart-PAP unless one is specifically prescribed.

The technology in this field is changing rapidly. If you are a candidate for CPAP, talk with the staff at your sleep center and with a homecare representative about the various versions of breathing devices that are available. You may want to test more than one and decide which one suits you best (see Chapter 13 for more on choosing a CPAP).

WHO CAN BENEFIT FROM USING CPAP?

CPAP can produce a virtual "miracle" cure in people who have not slept and breathed normally in years and are extremely ill from the cardiac and respiratory effects of years of sleep apnea. There are probably more than 2,500,000 people in the United States using CPAP today, with the numbers growing by the tens of thousands each year. However, many people have trouble adapting to the use of CPAP.

Treatment with CPAP should be started and evaluated in the sleep center during an overnight sleep study. This allows the sleep technician to adjust the pressure correctly, establish a baseline for monitoring the effectiveness of the treatment, and avoid inappropriate or ineffectual use of CPAP. In time, CPAPs may be able to accomplish this process accurately in the patient's home. However, that time has not yet arrived.

GETTING USED TO CPAP

The use of CPAP requires some motivation and perseverance. A few minutes are needed before going to bed each night to wash the face so the skin is clean and will not be irritated by the mask, and a few more minutes every morning to wash the mask. In addition, one simply needs to make a commitment to use the system each night for reasons of better health and longer life (see Chapsters 13 through 15 for more on using CPAP).

CPAP users generally are willing to put up with the inconvenience once they experience the results. In one follow-up study of 20 CPAP users after about a year, 16 were still using their CPAP all night, every night.[22] Such a high degree of compliance with the treatment reflects the users' enthusiasm for its effectiveness.

The main drawbacks of CPAP are related to its clumsiness, its effect on sleep, and its tendency to cause nasal irritation in some people. Some people can get used to wearing the mask in just one or two nights; others may take several weeks. The air pump motor makes a fanlike sound that a few CPAP users find to be too loud, but most do not object to it;

their bedmates generally find CPAP much easier to sleep with than explosive snoring.

People who use CPAP regularly occasionally stop using it for a while, but they generally return to it quickly because their apnea symptoms promptly return. In fact, after using CPAP and then sleeping without it, many people report that they had never been so aware of the choking they experienced with each apnea event. Now if they sleep without CPAP, they dream that heavy weights have been placed on their chest or they awaken feeling suffocated, so they are not often tempted to give up their CPAP.

When used all night, every night, CPAP provides positive results that are close to an instant cure. After beginning to use CPAP, most people report that within days they feel better than they have felt in many years. They report sleeping better, feeling rested in the morning and alert during the day, and having the energy to do the things they have been longing to do.

Please read Chapter 13 before you purchase a CPAP, and read Chapters 13 through 15 for suggestions on sleeping comfortably with a CPAP.

WHAT ARE THE LONG-TERM EFFECTS OF USING *CPAP?*

CPAP is a relatively recent development, having been in use in the United States only since about 1985. Sleep researchers have been watching carefully for any unfavorable long-term effects. By now many hundreds of people have been using CPAP for more than 10 years, and no serious negative consequences have been reported in the medical literature. Of course, no one can guarantee the safety of sleeping for 20 or 30 years under slightly higher air pressure, but so far the medical literature suggests that the long-term risks from sleep apnea are much more dangerous than the possibility of long-term risks from using CPAP.

HOW MUCH DO *CPAP* DEVICES COST?

CPAP systems can be obtained by rental or purchase. It is a good idea to begin by renting a system for two or three months, seeing how you do with it, and perhaps trying a couple of different models. Costs vary around the country. At the time of this writing, CPAP rentals cost approximately $200 per month, and the purchase price is in the neighborhood of $1,200. You may have to purchase the mask and tubing separately (about $130). The mask material tends to absorb oil from the skin and become stiff, so masks require periodic replacement (about $50). Older masks lasted only about six months, whereas newer silicone masks may last up to 18 months. A heated humidifier can cost $500, a nonheated one closer to $100.

Your health insurance may cover most, if not all, of the costs of CPAP. Talk to your insurance agent to find out which equipment and supplies they will cover (see Chapter 13 for more on selecting a CPAP).

How Can You Obtain a CPAP?

You must have a doctor's prescription to obtain a CPAP. Your sleep center personnel can put you in touch with a homecare company that will supply you with a CPAP system. The homecare company representative will send a respiratory therapist to your home to deliver the system and teach you how to operate it. They will provide same-day service in case of breakdown (see Chapters 13 and 14 on homecare companies).

A few sleep centers rent or sell CPAP systems directly. However, most do not have the desire or the staff to deal with the paperwork and home service that this involves.

Please read Chapter 13 before you purchase a CPAP, and read Chapters 14 and 15 for suggestions on sleeping comfortably with a CPAP.

OPAP™: Oral Pressure Appliance

Treating obstructive sleep apnea with a mouthpiece instead of a nose mask is a new idea. The OPAP (Figure 7.4) does just that. It is a small mouthpiece that can be worn either by itself or connected to CPAP tubing and a CPAP machine. By itself, the OPAP appliance can be used like a jaw retainer to hold the lower jaw in a forward position if desired. Attached to a CPAP, it holds the airway open with air pressure, just like a CPAP, but it uses the mouth instead of the nose.

WHO CAN BE HELPED BY AN *OPAP?*

The OPAP may be a new treatment choice for people with mild to severe obstructive sleep apnea who would otherwise be using a standard CPAP nose mask. It also is an option for people who have tried CPAP and had difficulty using it and for people who have had unsuccessful surgery for obstructive sleep apnea. Worn by itself, the OPAP may be an option for people who would otherwise use another of the dental appliances to treat obstructive sleep apnea. The advantage of the OPAP is that it bypasses the nose, where many people have nasal obstructions that make it difficult to use nasal CPAP. It also avoids the mask-fitting issues of CPAP and the skin irritation that some people experience from wearing the CPAP mask against the face. The OPAP does not require headgear, so it may be more comfortable, and it eliminates the "bad hair day" that can greet a person in the morning after wearing CPAP headgear all night.

WHAT ARE THE DRAWBACKS OF *OPAP?*

OPAP is so new that very few patients have had a chance to try it. We have not heard much direct feedback from patients about their satisfaction with an OPAP. In addition, long-term clinical effects are not yet available. Questions remain about how OPAP affects the teeth and the temporomandibular joint (TMJ). People with TMJ problems should consult their dentist about using an OPAP.

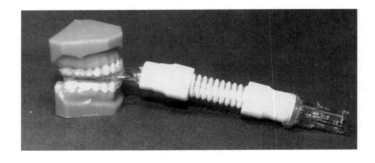

Figure 7.4

OPAP.

How Much Does an OPAP Cost?

At present an OPAP is custom fit like a dental appliance, which can be costly. The cost will probably be in the neighborhood of $500. A less expensive, off-the-shelf model may be available in the future. You should contact your insurance company if you are considering an OPAP and ask whether they will cover the cost.

How Can You Get an OPAP?

Ask your sleep specialist whether an OPAP would be appropriate for you. If so, he or she should be able to refer you to a dentist who is trained to fit an OPAP. If not, contact the Sleep Disorders Dental Society for the name of a dentist who is trained to treat sleep disorders.

Other Oral Appliances

A number of oral devices have been tried for treating sleep apnea. The objective of an oral device for sleep apnea is to hold the lower jaw, the tongue, or both, in a forward position during sleep. Theoretically, this should keep the airway open and prevent its collapse when the soft palate and tongue lose their muscle tone during sleep. Clearly, then, these devices are most likely to be effective for people whose obstructive apnea originates primarily in the lower pharynx (throat), by the position of their tongue or lower jaw in relation to their airway.

The Tongue-Retaining Device

The tongue-retaining device (TRD) is made of soft plastic and consists of a tongue-sized suction cup that is supposed to pull the tongue forward and hold it in that position. It is gripped by the teeth and held in place during sleep (Figure 7.5).

Many people who have used the TRD in experiments have found it moderately uncomfortable to wear. For this reason, it was worn only half the night in some experiments. Despite its drawbacks, the TRD was found to decrease the number of apnea events by approximately 50 percent. This means that the TRD could be about as effective as UPPP, a type of surgery described later.[23]

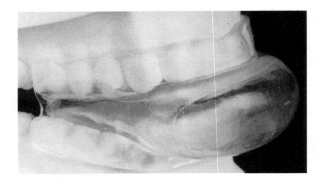

Figure 7.5

A Samelson-type tongue-retaining device. The tongue is drawn forward into the bubble and held by suction.

The TRD has not excited a lot of enthusiasm in the sleep research community, and so far it has not become widely used or available. Part of the reason for this probably is that the TRD apparently is useful only to a small group of obstructive apnea patients.

The people who are most likely to be helped by a TRD are those who are not obese, have no nasal obstructions, and have only mild to moderate apnea that is strongly influenced by sleeping position — that is, the apnea is much worse when sleeping on the back than when sleeping on the side.[24] For this group of people, apnea apparently is strongly affected by tongue position; therefore holding the tongue forward with the TRD is supposed to be helpful. In some cases more severe apnea has been controlled with the use of a TRD.

JAW RETAINERS

Another type of oral device that has been tested in several laboratories and sleep clinics is a jaw retainer, also called a *mandibular advancement device* (MAD). These are dental appliances that hold the lower jaw forward.[25,26]

Jaw retainers look like the bite plates or retainers that sometimes are prescribed by orthodontists. They are made of dental acrylic and may have metal loops over several teeth to hold the device in place (Figure 7.6).

Many different manufacturers have designed their own version of a jaw retainer. Some models are adjustable for easy selection of the best forward position for the lower jaw. Most jaw retainers must be custom-fitted.

Definitive studies to pinpoint who will benefit from a jaw retainer or which devices work best have not been completed. Studies of mandibular appliances in sleep apnea patients have used small numbers of patients and different definitions of "success." So far these limited clinical trials suggest that mandibular devices are about 50 percent effective. That is, about 50 percent of patients who try them still have serious enough sleep apnea symptoms that they need additional treatment. The adjustable models may be more practical than models that are not adjustable. It is unlikely that any one design will work equally well for all patients.

For these and other reasons, people who are considering an oral appliances would be wise to consult a dentist who is experienced in using these devices and who works in cooperation with a sleep specialist. The sleep specialist (not the dentist) should make the diagnosis of obstructive sleep apnea and should measure the effectiveness of the dental device after the dentist has fit the patient with it. You can locate a dentist near you who has been trained in this field by contacting the Sleep Disorders Dental Society (see Appendix).

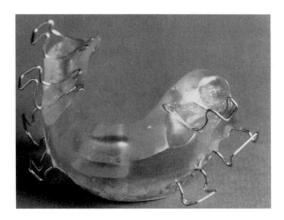

Figure 7.6
A typical example of a jaw-retaining device. The metal loops hold the lower jaw in a forward position.

Who Can Benefit from Using a Jaw Retainer?

The manufacturers of jaw retainers and some experimenters who have patients using them have reported some good results, especially in patients who have mild to moderate apnea.[26–29]

Because jaw-retaining devices concentrate their treatment on the lower jaw and/or tongue, people with a smallish lower jaw that is set somewhat far back (called by orthodontists a class II occlusion) are likely to have good results.

Retainers also have been used successfully in children born with irregularly formed jaws who have difficulty with obstructive apnea.

Three-quarters of people with sleep apnea have airway obstructions in more than one place. People whose obstructive apnea results mostly from nasal problems or from the upper pharynx (large tonsils, adenoids, soft palate, uvula) are not likely to be treated successfully with an oral device and will need further treatment. In fact, you must be able to breathe through your nose to use the retainer; a person with a nasal obstruction or a stuffy nose from an allergy or a cold will be unable to wear one. Even some people who seem likely candidates for a jaw retainer continue to have apnea events, as shown by heavy snoring. Also, it is necessary to have an adequate number of teeth to be able to hold an appliance in place.

One group of people who may want to try an oral appliance are those who have been unable to use CPAP despite a wholehearted effort. If a nasal obstruction is preventing you from successfully using CPAP, it also will prevent you from using an oral appliance. If you can eliminate the nasal obstruction (by surgery or medication), you may then be able to use CPAP.

There may be a place for occasional use of an oral device, even if it is only partially effective, for example:

1. When CPAP is unavailable (backpacking, primitive travel);

2. When the device allows the patient to use a lower CPAP pressure; and

3. When screening patients for mandibular advancement surgery (to simulate the possible results of surgery).

Objective studies of the benefit in these situations are not yet available.

Getting Used to a Jaw Retainer

It may take from several nights to several weeks to get completely accustomed to wearing a jaw retainer. Excess saliva will probably be an early side effect. Any foreign object in the mouth, such as a retainer, causes the production of excess saliva at first, but this generally tapers off after a night or two. However, it may take as long as two or three weeks for jaw muscles and other muscles to become accustomed to wearing a retainer. The retainer may need to be worn that long to carry out a fair trial of the device and decide whether it is effective.

A disadvantage of the jaw retainer is that you cannot rent one to try it out. One "do-it-yourself" brand, which is available by prescription, can be adapted to fit by warming it in hot water. It works well enough to offer some idea of effectiveness, but it is not very durable. Otherwise, you will not know whether a jaw retainer works for you until you have paid to have one made. If it does work, you will be delighted. A jaw-retaining device is less restrictive of movement, much smaller, less expensive, and more convenient to deal with than a breathing device. If it does not work, other options are available.

How Much Do Jaw Retainers Cost?

Jaw retainers are less expensive than CPAP units, but still surprisingly expensive. The do-it-yourself brand costs about $25. Some sleep centers have trained technicians who can fit an adjustable model for $300 to $400. Some manufacturers charge as much as $600 for a custom-fitted appliance, and with the dentist's markup it may cost you more than $1,000. That is approximately twice the cost of an ordinary orthodontic retainer and does not include the cost of having your orthodontist or dentist take jaw impressions, or the cost of additional visits to check or adjust the fit of the appliance. This can add another several hundred dollars to the cost. Check with your insurance company in advance to see if they will cover part or all of these costs.

Should You Try a Jaw Retainer?

If you and your sleep specialist think you are a likely candidate for success with a jaw retainer, here are some questions to answer:

1. Have you had a sleep study to measure the baseline of your sleep apnea before treatment?

2. Is your sleep apnea mild?

3. If your sleep apnea is moderate to severe, have you tried CPAP (a more effective treatment)?

4. Do you have nasal obstructions that would prevent you from breathing through your nose?

5. Do you have temporomandibular joint (TMJ) syndrome or dental problems that might be aggravated by using a jaw retainer?

6. If you have TMJ or dental problems, can your sleep specialist refer you to a dentist who is experienced in fitting oral appliances for sleep apnea?

7. Has your sleep specialist scheduled you for a follow-up sleep study while you are wearing the oral appliance to verify its effectiveness?

8. Have you added up and talked with your insurance agent about the full costs of an oral device, including fabrication, fitting, office visits for adjustments, and a follow-up sleep test? Do you consider this a cost-effective treatment option?

These questions are based partly on standards suggested by the American Academy of Sleep Medicine for the use of oral appliances.[30]

IS THE ORAL APPLIANCE REALLY WORKING?

Soon after you become accustomed to using an oral appliance, you should return to the sleep center for a follow-up sleep study to determine whether the appliance is effectively eliminating your apnea. The sleep study must assess whether the retainer works both when you are sleeping on your back and when you are sleeping on your side.

Drugs for Treating Obstructive Sleep Apnea

So far drugs generally have not been shown to be very effective in treating obstructive sleep apnea. However, several of the drugs that have been tried unsuccessfully as treatments for central apnea (described previously) have met with at least mixed success in obstructive apnea.

The hormone *medroxyprogesterone* has been found to be somewhat effective in some people with the Pickwickian syndrome (see Chapter 8). It has been reported to improve the breathing drive, to decrease the number of apnea events, and to improve the patient's symptoms.[8,31,32] However, some researchers have reported no improvement in apneas, so the results with this drug are conflicting.[6,8,32]

Medroxyprogesterone has some undesirable side effects. It can cause fluid retention, nausea, and depression in some people. Because it is a sex hormone, it may cause extra hair growth and breast tenderness. It should not be used by people with blood-clotting disorders or liver disease, by pregnant women, or by people known or suspected to have genital cancer.

Protriptyline is an antidepressant that is variably effective in mild cases of sleep apnea. It is only a treatment option if the person's life is not in immediate danger from the effects of sleep apnea.

Drawbacks of protriptyline are that it decreases the amount of REM sleep and has a high incidence of other side effects, including dry mouth, constipation (mild to intolerable), difficulty starting urine flow, and impotence.[31,33] It can cause confusion, especially in elderly people. It may be contraindicated (an undesirable treatment choice) for people with arrhythmias, very high blood pressure, glaucoma, or prostate disease.[32]

Oxygen alone is not an effective treatment for obstructive sleep apnea; in fact, it can make obstructive apnea worse.

Other drugs have been tried as treatment for obstructive sleep apnea but have not been found to be effective.

Surgery for Obstructive Sleep Apnea

Surgery is the least conservative treatment for obstructive sleep apnea. It would be wise to understand the other alternatives before selecting this one.

Four general types of surgery are used to treat obstructive sleep apnea:

- Nasal surgery
- Palate and tongue surgeries
  - UPPP (uvulopalatopharyngoplasty)
  - LAUP (laser-assisted uvulopalatoplasty for snoring)
  - Somnoplasty™ (radiofrequency thermal ablation)
- Jaw surgery and other maxillofacial surgeries
- Tracheostomy

NASAL SURGERY

Nasal surgery actually may refer to several different ear, nose, and throat (ENT) procedures. These can include repair of the nasal septum (the wall that separates your left and right nasal passages), turbinate surgery to remove bony obstructions, removal of polyps, surgery on the nasal sinuses, or submucous resection (removing loose tissue under the lining of the nasal passages).

Nasal surgery may be a necessary first step for some people to allow them to use CPAP. People with nasal obstructions may feel "claustrophobic" or suffocated while using CPAP, or they may unconsciously pull off the CPAP mask during sleep. CPAP users who have these problems should talk with their sleep specialist about whether nasal surgery might make them more comfortable with CPAP.

Nasal surgery may also permit a person to wear an oral appliance that would have been impossible before surgery. A person who has poor airflow through his nose would feel suffocated wearing an oral appliance in his mouth.

By itself, nasal surgery usually is not an effective treatment for sleep apnea or snoring. Some people occasionally report a decrease in snoring after surgery on their nose, only to have the symptoms return over several months.

However, improved airflow through the nose can have a significant effect on overall airflow, and it should also be considered as part of an overall surgical approach if palate surgery (see the next section) is going to be carried out.

PALATE AND TONGUE SURGERIES

Uvulopalatopharyngoplasty

Uvulopalatopharyngoplasty (UPPP) has been the most common type of surgery for sleep apnea. Under general anesthesia, a scalpel is used to remove approximately the rear third of the soft palate. The back of the soft palate is left in a streamlined shape that will be less likely to collapse during sleep (Figure 7.7).

Who Can Be Helped by UPPP? Whether a person can be helped by UPPP depends on the reason for surgery and on how one defines being "helped." If the surgery is for purely "cosmetic" purposes (i.e., *simply to cut down on snoring*) and if a sleep study has shown that the person has *only* snoring and *not* sleep apnea, UPPP stands about a 90 percent chance of being successful. The bedmate's report that snoring has disappeared after UPPP does not necessarily mean the disappearance of sleep apnea.

If the purpose of surgery is to eliminate sleep apnea, the chance of success is much lower and much more difficult to predict. In this case, the decision to have surgery is best reached after extensive discussion of the operation and the expected results with your sleep specialist and ENT surgeon.

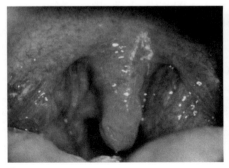 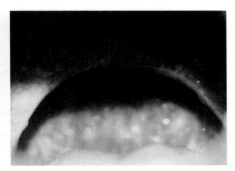

A   B

Figure 7.7

UPPP surgery:
(A) Before. Notice the large tonsils and fleshy uvula.
(B) After. Tonsils and uvula have been removed.

It is important to distinguish between an attempt to *help* sleep apnea and an attempt to *cure* sleep apnea (i.e., eliminate all disease). Uvulo-palatopharyngoplasty surgery can *help* sleep apnea to varying degrees in different people. For example, Patients A and B might both show significant improvement after surgery. However, Patient A might have started out with mild apnea and may not need further treatment despite some remaining sleep apnea. (An example would be a person who goes from a sleepy patient with a respiratory disturbance index (RDI) of 40 before surgery to an alert patient with an RDI of 10 after UPPP.) Patient B, on the other hand, might have started with more serious apnea and may need further treatment after UPPP. (An example would be a person whose RDI of 60 improves to 30 after surgery but who still has low blood oxygen at night and is still drowsy.)

How often is sleep apnea *cured* by UPPP? That is difficult to say, but probably less than 20 percent of the time. Results like those of Patient A, who needs no further treatment, probably account for 20 percent to 40 percent of UPPP cases. People like Patient B, who needs treatment after surgery, probably account for 50 percent to 70 percent of UPPP cases.

People who are the most likely candidates for success with this type of surgery meet the following criteria:

1. They are not more than 25 percent or 30 percent over their ideal weight, and they do not gain weight after surgery.[34,35]

2. They have only slight to moderate apnea, and it is all obstructive apnea.

3. Their apnea arises mostly from some obvious anatomic obstruction of the upper part of the pharynx (throat) — the soft palate or upper throat area.[36,37] This includes people with enlarged tonsils or adenoids (tonsils and adenoids often are removed during UPPP); people with a very long soft palate or a large, fleshy uvula; and people with excess fleshy tissue in the throat region.

In contrast, people with very severe apnea or those whose apnea arises from places other than the area of the soft palate are not good candidates for UPPP. Those with a lower jaw that is very short or placed far back, or with a tongue that is positioned fairly far back and low in the neck, or with apnea arising in the lower pharynx are less likely to be successful with UPPP.[37,38]

Weight gain is an extremely important factor in the success of UPPP. The extra loading of the abdomen, which interferes with the breathing reflex, plus the fatty deposits in the neck, which help obstruct the airway, can overpower any positive results that may be gained from UPPP. Therefore, people who have UPPP and then gain weight are likely to see the return of obstructive apnea.[34]

Until recently, not much was known about which people could best be helped by UPPP. With the aid of cephalometry (measurement of size and placement of structures in the head using radiographs, CAT scan, or MRI pictures) and fiberoptic examination of the inside of the airway, doctors are gradually gaining more information about how to choose the most likely candidates for successful UPPP.[38,42] Nevertheless, no one can accurately predict the success of UPPP.

Determining whether you are a good candidate for UPPP must be done by consulting your sleep expert and a good otolaryngologist (ENT specialist) who has experience not only with eliminating snoring but also with sleep apnea problems. The otolaryngologist should examine your throat internally. He may order a radiograph, MRI, or CAT scan of your head so that he can measure the sizes and relationships between various anatomic features that cause your obstructive apnea. This will help him determine your chances of being helped by UPPP.

What Are the Drawbacks to Uvulopalatopharyngoplasty? Compared with many surgical procedures, uvulopalatopharyngoplasty is not a particularly risky kind of surgery. It does not involve any large arteries or nerves. It may be performed as outpatient surgery in healthy, uncomplicated cases. A hospital stay of one or two days may be necessary for some patients.

As mentioned previously, the greatest risk probably is from the anesthesia. The more narrow the airway, the greater the risk from preoperative medications, from anesthetics, and from painkillers and sedatives given immediately after the operation.[1]

The reason for this increased risk is that anesthetics and some other drugs interfere with the breathing reflexes. If you have sleep apnea, you already have breathing reflexes that may not operate quite normally. This means that you are at somewhat greater than normal risk from anesthesia. This breathing abnormality, coupled with existing apnea, possible throat obstruction from postoperative swelling, and perhaps pain medication could add up to serious complications.

Pain is another consideration with UPPP. People who have had UPPP report that the pain after the operation is very severe — more painful than expected (e.g., more painful than a tonsillectomy). Severe pain can last as long as a week.

All patients report difficulty with swallowing after surgery. The removal of the uvula at the back of the mouth cavity makes it easier for material from the mouth to be pushed up into the back of the nasal cavity during swallowing. This is a common problem for the first two weeks after surgery, but it should correct itself with time, particularly if the surgeon is skilled and experienced with the procedure. A few people continue to have swallowing problems. However, most who do have a little difficulty swallowing find that they overcome the problem with some practice and if they eat properly.[1,35]

There have been reports of airway obstruction becoming worse or more difficult to treat with CPAP following UPPP.

Why Have Uvulopalatopharyngoplasty If the Odds Are Poor? Even if the chances of being helped enough not to require further treatment are 50 percent to 60 percent, you may prefer taking a chance in the hope of avoiding other treatments, such as CPAP, oral appliances, or other surgeries.

UPPP has a very low risk when performed on patients who have been carefully tested at a good sleep center, and when the surgery is performed by an experienced ENT surgeon. (For example, at Providence Medical Center in Seattle there never has been a surgical fatality or serious complication.)

How Can You Arrange for Uvulopalatopharyngoplasty? It is not wise to have UPPP as a treatment for sleep apnea until you have been thoroughly examined by a physician who understands the causes of sleep apnea and knows how to weigh the benefits against the risks in your particular case. The sleep specialist, in turn, can refer you to a surgeon who is experienced with UPPP if you appear to be a good candidate for successful treatment by this procedure.

Laser Surgery to Treat Snoring

Laser-assisted uvulopalatoplasty (LAUP) is a newer technique for surgery on the soft palate that has been promoted recently as a harmless way to eliminate simple snoring. However, snoring is a symptom of sleep apnea, and in definitive studies LAUP has *not* been shown to be an effective treatment for sleep apnea.[43,44]

The distinction between simple snoring and sleep apnea is not always clear. People who appear to have "simple snoring" frequently turn out to have significant sleep apnea.[43] LAUP surgeons often try to screen out those patients with a questionnaire on snoring. However, questionnaires cannot accurately diagnose sleep apnea and tend to underestimate it. Consequently, many patients with undiagnosed sleep apnea have had LAUP surgery and have been left with a serious underlying disorder. To avoid unnecessary, possibly harmful LAUP surgery, people who snore should first be evaluated by a sleep specialist to rule out sleep apnea. Only after sleep apnea has been ruled out should people consider LAUP.

LAUP has been promoted as a substitute for conventional palate surgery (i.e., UPPP, as described previously). Patients whose sleep and ENT specialists consider them good candidates for UPPP for treatment of snoring may want to consider LAUP for this purpose, but not to treat sleep apnea.

What Is LAUP? LAUP involves several lengthwise laser "cuts" making a V-shaped pattern on the soft palate. Several sessions usually are needed. The laser cauterizes ("cooks") the tissue, leaving narrow scars that stiffen the tissue and presumably diminish the vibration that causes snoring.

Does LAUP Eliminate Snoring? Proponents claim that it does in 80 percent to 90 percent of cases, but there are reports that snoring may return within two years after surgery in some cases.[45]

How Does LAUP Compare with Conventional UPPP? LAUP is less risky — it involves less time, less bleeding, less tissue removal, no general anesthetic, and no hospitalization. It is somewhat less expensive (expect charges of approximately $1,600 for surgeon, plus an additional fee for the surgical facility). Conventional UPPP involves a general anesthetic; possibly a hospital stay; significant pain; and risks from bleeding, infection, and general anesthetic. UPPP may cost up to $3,000.

Please read the sections in this chapter on choosing surgery in general and on UPPP.

Can LAUP Cure Sleep Apnea? No, it cannot, according to analyses published to date.[43] LAUP may be helpful as an adjunct treatment for mild to moderate apnea, with approximately 50 percent of patients obtaining 50 percent or better improvement. Careful examination of the airway may identify people who are likely to have poor results. These include patients with a large tongue and a small palate.

The main danger from LAUP is that people who have a potentially fatal disorder, sleep apnea, may have LAUP under the mistaken impression that the surgery will cure them. Sleep apnea is more than snoring (see Chapter 4, "What Causes Sleep Apnea?").

The American Academy of Sleep Medicine's standards of practice for LAUP recommend that patients be evaluated by a sleep specialist before having LAUP. People with sleep apnea should have a follow-up sleep study after surgery to determine whether the sleep apnea has been eliminated.[44]

Somnoplasty™ (Radiofrequency Surgical Ablation)

Somnoplasty is another new technique. It uses radiofrequency energy to shrink the bulk of soft tissue. In 1998 the U.S. Food and Drug Administration (FDA) approved Somnoplasty on the upper airway (e.g., soft palate and base of tongue) for treatment of sleep apnea.

Like LAUP, Somnoplasty is being promoted to the general public as a simple solution for the common, desperately annoying problem of snoring. As with LAUP, patients run the risk of bypassing an important medical issue — undiagnosed sleep apnea.

Like LAUP, Somnoplasty by itself does *not* appear to be an effective treatment for moderate to severe sleep apnea. It may be helpful in milder cases, perhaps in combination with other treatments such as CPAP, weight loss, or an oral appliance. Definitive controlled studies on Somnoplasty have not yet been published.

How Does Somnoplasty Work? Somnoplasty uses high-frequency radio waves to destroy cells by heating, causing the formation of a scar. The scar shrinks and reduces the bulk of the tissue. A crude version of this technology has been used for years in surgery to cauterize bleeding capillaries and to eliminate small tumors. In the case of Somnoplasty, a much lower level of energy is used.

The procedure is performed in the doctor's office. The operator anesthetizes the area and then inserts a thin electrode into the tissue. The electrode emits radiofrequency energy that creates a lesion; basically the energy "cooks" a small area of tissue. Each lesion takes three to six minutes to create, and several lesions usually are made during a single session.

Swelling occurs within the few days after the surgical session, and scar tissue replaces the lesions within a couple of weeks. The scarring shrinks the area and decreases the bulk of the tissue. The amount of the decrease depends on the amount of scarring produced.[46]

Two to four surgical sessions are reported to be needed for best results, with eight weeks for healing between sessions.

What Are the Risks from Somnoplasty? Because Somnoplasty requires only a local rather than a general anesthetic, it may involve fewer surgical risks than scalpel surgery. No significant side effects had been reported after one year of experience with Somnoplasty. Long-term results are not yet known.

Swelling occurs after the surgery, which can be risky for sleep apnea patients who have difficulty keeping their airway open. Patients should sleep at a 45-degree angle after surgery while they still have some swelling.

A risk that Somnoplasty shares with LAUP is that it silences the major warning sign of sleep apnea by eliminating snoring, and patients can be left to unknowingly suffer the long-term effects of an undiagnosed, potentially harmful disorder.

Another potential risk with Somnoplasty relates to the training and experience of the person performing the operation. If you are considering Somnoplasty, you would be wise to ask about the medical qualifications of the individual who will be performing the actual procedure.

Can Palate Somnoplasty Effectively Treat Sleep Apnea? In palate surgery by Somnoplasty, a series of lesions are created in the soft palate over the course of three or four surgical sessions, with the goal of shrinking and tightening the palate.

The FDA has approved the use of Somnoplasty on the upper airway (palate, tongue) as a treatment for sleep apnea. *However, it is unlikely to be more effective than LAUP or UPPP for apnea because it affects the same tissue. Long-term results are not yet available.*

A reputable Somnoplasty practitioner will ask you whether you have symptoms of sleep apnea, counsel you about its possible dangers, and refer you for appropriate sleep testing. If this does not happen, and if you have underlying sleep apnea, do not count on a cure from Somnoplasty.

It is extremely important to return to your sleep specialist and have a sleep study following Somnoplasty to find out whether your sleep apnea has been eliminated, even if you feel that it has.

Does Palate Somnoplasty Eliminate Snoring? Reports suggest that it can decrease or eliminate snoring about as well as LAUP. Long-term results are not yet available.

Tongue Reduction by Somnoplasty In tongue reduction by Somnoplasty,[47] the goal is to decrease the bulk of the tongue so it does not obstruct the throat. In the past, a scalpel or laser was used to remove a notch of tissue at the back of the tongue, sometimes along with some tonsil tissue that is located at the base of the tongue.[48] Because Somnoplasty is such a new technique, no one knows whether this type of surgery on the tongue will be more or less effective than the laser method, so results are difficult to predict.

The success of tongue reduction surgery in treating apnea also is difficult to predict. Two groups of surgeons reported the results of laser tongue surgery on 24 patients who had already had unsuccessful UPPP surgery.[48,49] Following laser tongue surgery, fewer than than half of the procedures were considered "successful," and those patients still had an average RDI above 10 and blood oxygen levels below 90, which means that many of them would still end up on CPAP. Tongue Somnoplasty is still an experimental procedure, but shows some promise as a treatment for obstructive sleep apnea.

How Does Somnoplasty Compare with LAUP and Conventional UPPP? Somnoplasty is less risky than UPPP, involving less bleeding, no hospitalization, and no general anesthetic. According to one published report, Somnoplasty is less painful than LAUP during recovery. The cost of Somnoplasty currently is $1,600 to $2,000 and usually is not paid for by insurance.

JAW SURGERY AND OTHER MAXILLOFACIAL SURGERIES

Maxillofacial surgery is surgery on the mandible (lower jaw) and the other bones and tissue of the face. Head and neck surgery involves the other parts of the head, face, and airway, and is performed by otolaryngologists, or ENTs. These surgeries are not new, but they have a fairly short history of use as a treatment for sleep apnea, so in a sense they should be considered somewhat experimental. These surgeries include:

- Mandibular advancement — moves the lower jaw forward
- Midface advancement — moves the upper jaw forward
- Hyoid surgery — repositions the base of the tongue

Jaw surgery and other maxillofacial surgeries for treating sleep apnea actually include a half dozen possible surgical procedures and many variations. All are aimed at eliminating obstructions in the airway between the lower jaw and the back of the throat.

Several different techniques are used to move the tongue forward by surgery on the jaw. The procedure may range from moving a small rectangular piece of bone from the tip of the jaw to moving the entire jaw by cutting through it on both sides.

Other surgical procedures reposition the hyoid bone at the base of the tongue. These are fairly new and still experimental (Figure 7.8). A surgical team at Stanford that has pioneered this surgery now performs a two-stage procedure involving UPPP, tongue advancement, and hyoid suspension, followed by upper/lower jaw advancement.[50]

Who Can Be Helped by Jaw Surgery and Other Maxillofacial Surgeries? It is not yet possible to predict precisely who will be helped by these surgeries. More experience is needed with this type of surgery as a treatment for sleep apnea before such predictions can be made with assurance. Many factors may influence the outcome, including not only the structure of the skull and soft tissue, but also obesity, age, neuro-muscular control of the airway, the presence of other sleep disorders, and, of course, the skill and experience of the surgical team.

Mandibular advancement is the simplest and safest of these proce-dures and is being used more often nationally, although its usefulness has not yet been fully established. It has been used only in a relatively small number of patients with complicated apnea. An example is one patient who had a very small jaw and a small airway opening and for whom neither UPPP nor medication had helped. In this case, surgery did not completely eliminate his apnea, but it cut it by approximately half.[51] As with many examples of sleep apnea surgery, whether the results are successful depends on if you define "success" as complete elimination of the apnea or if you are satisfied with elimination of half of the apnea.

Among 1,000 people with obstructive apnea studied at one sleep center, about 6 percent had an obviously malformed lower jaw, and another 32 percent had a slightly short lower jaw.[52] It is among these people that the best candidates for mandibular advancement surgery would probably be found, because their apnea is likely to arise in part from structural problems in the lower pharynx — a jaw and tongue positioned further back and lower than normal and an unusually small lower airway opening.

These complicated surgeries for sleep apnea should be planned as a team effort, involving the sleep specialist, an ENT specialist, the max-

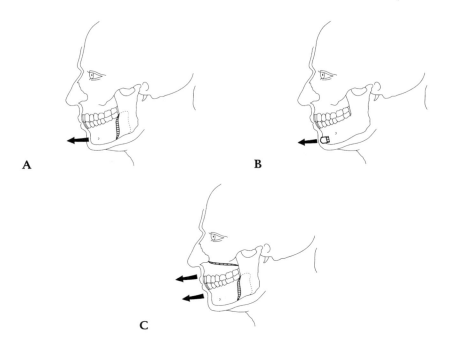

Figure 7.8

Examples of mandibular and maxillofacial surgeries that have been tried for treating obstructive sleep apnea:
(A) and (B), two ways of pulling the lower jaw and the base of the tongue forward.
(C) Moving both the upper and lower jaw forward.

illofacial surgeon who will perform the actual mandibular surgery, and an orthodontist if teeth are to be repositioned.[52]

The surgery itself is fairly safe if it is performed by an experienced surgeon. It is, however, performed under general anesthesia, which, as noted previously, is especially risky for people with breathing disorders.

What Are the Drawbacks to Maxillofacial Surgery? One major problem that may arise is difficulty with the healing of the jawbone because the blood supply to that area is not very generous. If the jaw is cut on both sides and moved forward (sliding osteotomy), the jaw may be wired closed during healing for about six weeks, which presents a significant inconvenience to the patient. In addition, orthodontics may also be required to reposition the teeth and realign the bite. The entire procedure is expensive and time-consuming.

Another important drawback with this surgery should be considered. After mandibular surgery, the jawbone has a tendency to reposition itself backward again toward its original location. This happens over the course of several years in response to the powerful force of the tongue muscles, which are constantly pulling on the jawbone. Although some surgeons would disagree, other physicians have serious doubts about how long the results of this type of surgery will last.

TRACHEOSTOMY

Tracheostomy used to be a standard treatment for sleep apnea, but it has become much less common since the advent of CPAP. Today it is performed primarily on two types of patients: people who are very sick from the effects of sleep apnea and who need immediate (sometimes emergency) treatment to save their lives, and those for whom other treatments have been unsuccessful. Tracheostomy has become the treatment of last resort; if all else fails, tracheostomy can be counted on to eliminate sleep apnea. In that sense, it is a very hopeful form of surgery. It also is fairly simple.

What Is a Tracheostomy? In a tracheostomy, a small opening is made into the trachea (windpipe), in the front of the neck just below the larynx (voice box). This opening may be considered permanent if tracheostomy is to be the permanent method of treating the person's sleep apnea. The opening can be surgically closed sometime in the future, if, for example, the patient switches to CPAP or some other therapy. The idea of a tracheostomy is to allow air to bypass the obstructions in the upper airway. The tracheostomy opening is closed with a plug during waking hours, and the person breathes normally through his nose and mouth. At night, however, the tracheostomy is left open, and breathing is done through the neck opening, unobstructed.

A tracheostomy tube usually is worn in the tracheostomy opening. This is a small, curved tube with a flange at the top. It is inserted through the tracheostomy opening and extends several inches down into the windpipe. The tracheostomy tube usually is worn permanently.

The flange at the top helps hold the tube in place and protects the opening in the throat (Figure 7.9).

Tracheostomy surgery itself is not particularly risky, although it usually is done under general anesthesia, which may be risky.

Complications that may arise with tracheostomy fall into two categories. One involves the tracheostomy opening itself. In some cases the opening tries to close itself up again. Other difficulties can result if the tissue around the opening heals incorrectly or becomes infected, damaged, or eroded. Several different surgical variations have been developed in an attempt to avoid such problems. One variation is called a flap tracheostomy, in which the opening in the throat is lined with skin. This is intended to eliminate the need for a tracheostomy tube.

Another set of complications of tracheostomy is respiratory infections such as pneumonia. When a person is breathing through a tracheostomy, he virtually is breathing straight into his lungs, bypassing all the natural germ-filtering systems in his nose and upper airway. Consequently, bacteria, viruses, and other foreign objects can much more easily reach the lungs. Great care must be taken to prevent this from happening.

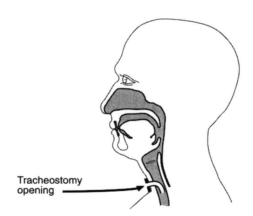

Tracheostomy
opening

Figure 7.9
A tracheostomy, with tube in place. At night, the patient breathes through the tracheostomy opening, bypassing the obstruction in his airway. During the day, the tube is closed with a plug, so that the patient can talk.

There may be a fair amount of pain, some swelling, and difficulty swallowing for several days after tracheostomy surgery. Even after flap tracheostomy, a tracheostomy tube is worn until the incision has healed. The tube is chosen for size and shape to fit the particular person and is not particularly uncomfortable to wear.

The patient and his family, and eventually the patient himself, need to follow a fairly rigorous, 24-hour postoperative program of taking care of the tracheostomy. This includes cleaning, suctioning, misting, and applying salt solution and antibiotics. Immediately after surgery, a suction machine must be used periodically to keep the trach tube clear of mucous secretions that could block the airway. The suction machine will be needed indefinitely for cleaning the tube and preventing mucous buildup. Mucous production decreases as time goes on, so the frequency of suctioning also decreases. A humidifier can be used at night for the first several weeks after surgery to help keep mucous secretions from drying and blocking the tube. Cleanliness will continue to be extremely important at all times to avoid introducing bacteria into the tracheostomy opening. The nurses and respiratory therapists should be explicit in teaching all these procedures to both patient and family.

Who Can Be Helped by a Tracheostomy? Anyone with obstructive or mixed sleep apnea can be helped by a tracheostomy. Nowadays the people chosen for tracheostomy usually have severe apnea with severe complications, including excessive daytime drowsiness, such that they are completely disabled.[53] They may have tried other treatments and found them unsuccessful. They may have significant cardiac arrhythmias or other serious heart complications from severe sleep apnea. They may have extremely low oxygen levels in their blood.

Tracheostomy eliminates snoring, improves the quality of sleep, and virtually cures daytime drowsiness and apnea in nearly everyone who has the surgery. It greatly improves fatigue and morning headaches.[53]

What Are the Drawbacks to Tracheostomy? One of the main drawbacks of tracheostomy, and one reason it has fallen out of favor so quickly with the advent of CPAP, is the impact that it has on day-to-day lifestyle.

Most people need several weeks to months to learn to deal with the frustrations of tracheostomy hygiene and to adjust to their new image with a tracheostomy opening in the throat. A bout of depression commonly accompanies this adjustment period. The severity and duration of the person's depression (in fact, whether it occurs at all) depend on the individual, on how well the person has been prepared for the appearance and the care of the tracheostomy, and on family support. The patient, spouse, and other close family members should be counseled about the surgical procedure, the care that is necessary afterward, and the likelihood of temporary depression. Talking with other people who have tracheostomies and are attending sleep apnea support groups, both before and after surgery, helps people to adjust more easily.

Most people who have had tracheostomies report that they do just fine once the initial adjustment period is over. They lead normal, active lives and generally do not seem to be bothered by their tracheostomies. However, they will always have to be careful about hygiene around the tracheostomy opening. And they must always take care that nothing enters the windpipe through the tracheostomy opening. For example, people with tracheostomies may not swim. Because the opening in the throat leads almost directly into the lungs, people with tracheostomies are in extreme danger from drowning and therefore must avoid not only swimming but also all water-related activities (water skiing, sailing, rafting, fishing from a boat) that might require swimming.

Other drawbacks involve the cosmetics of covering the tracheostomy opening. A small plate or shield is worn over the opening and is held in place by a cord around the neck (Figure 7.10). There is nothing inherently objectionable about its appearance, but many people choose to cover the tracheostomy plate with a turtleneck or a scarf. On some people the opening is a little too high to be easily covered by clothing. One such patient recommended making a high-necked, elastic-topped dickey.[54]

Another problem can be keeping the opening sealed during the day. Talking becomes difficult if there is air leakage. Coughing or sneezing

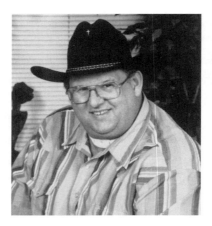

Figure 7.10
This person has a tracheostomy.

can sometimes pop the seal and cause temporary embarrassment.

Other difficulties are problems that can arise from poor healing or erosion of the opening. To avoid such problems, it pays to find the most skillful surgeon you can (consider a plastic surgeon) and to carefully follow the postoperative instructions. Ask your doctor to answer any questions you may have and be persistent in asking for help in learning to deal with any follow-up problems.

WEIGHT LOSS SURGERY (GASTRIC BYPASS)

Weight loss surgery has been called "behavioral surgery"[55] because it surgically enforces a change in a person's eating behavior that the person has been unable to accomplish by other means. The desired change in behavior is to reduce the amount of food the person consumes at any one sitting. This is done surgically by making the stomach smaller.

Several versions of weight loss surgery have been tried over the past 20 years. The most common procedure performed today is gastric bypass, in which the stomach is reduced in size, not by removing part of the stomach, but by placing a row of staples across it, dividing the stomach into a small upper pouch and a larger lower pouch. The upper pouch becomes the "new" stomach. It receives food from the esophagus and empties into a branch of the intestines that has been brought up and attached to it.

After surgery, food intake at any one time will always be restricted to approximately twice the volume of the "new" stomach, which usually is about 30 ml. This means that no more than about one-quarter of a cup of food can be eaten at a time.

Gastric bypass is major surgery (Figure 7.11). It involves major organs (stomach and intestines), some large arteries, and the opening and closing of the abdominal cavity. There are risks from anesthesia and other medications. During and after surgery the placement of a number of tubes will add further to the invasiveness of the procedure: a nasogastric tube for removing fluid from the stomach, catheters, intravenous hookups, and possibly an endotracheal tube for a ventilator. Gastric bypass surgery requires a hospital stay of a week or more, considerable postoperative pain and discomfort, and an extended recovery period lasting from four to five weeks to months.

Additional risk factors arise because this surgery is performed on obese people. The possibility of death from surgery is two to three times greater for obese people than for people of average weight.[55] Consequently, it is important to carefully weigh the risks against the possible

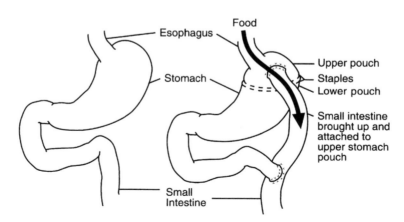

Figure 7.11

Gastric bypass surgery: the stomach is stapled crossways, which greatly reduces the amount of food it can hold. A loop of small intestine is attached to the upper stomach pouch to receive its contents.

benefits that can reasonably be anticipated after surgery.

Complications after bypass surgery can be significant. They may include infections, bowel obstruction, collapse of lungs, blood clots, and other after-effects seen following abdominal surgery. (Obese people also have about twice the rate of postoperative complications compared with people of ideal weight.) The most common complication after gastric bypass is excessive vomiting.[55]

Who Can Be Helped by Gastric Bypass?

People who undergo gastric bypass usually are characterized as being "morbidly obese." The average weight of 17 patients in one group was twice their recommended body weight.[56] They are *not* people who are having cosmetic surgery to lose weight; they are people whose lives are in danger because of their excessive weight and other complications.

The patients chosen for gastric bypass usually are screened to include only those who have already attempted to lose weight under carefully supervised weight loss programs. The patient's psychological status often is evaluated as part of the screening process. Patients should understand the risks and behavioral changes that will be necessary for the bypass surgery to be successful.

How Effective Is Gastric Bypass in Treating Apnea?

One study reported that most of their patients' sleep apnea was significantly improved six months after surgery. Some patients had completely lost their symptoms. Many patients reported no daytime sleepiness or loud snoring. Changes in personality also were reported — greater responsiveness, fewer emotional problems, less difficulty at work. A full year is needed for complete results, so during the six months following that report the patients in the study group might anticipate additional weight loss and further improvement in their apnea symptoms.[56] In the long term, however, some people who have had gastric bypass surgery will return to their presurgery weight. The overall failure rate for gastric bypass surgery is reported to be from 30 percent to 50 percent.[55]

In summary, gastric bypass surgery may be an effective and permanent — if radical — solution for severely obese apnea patients who are motivated to change their eating behavior. The possible benefits should be carefully weighed against the significant potential risks.

Mr. Kennedy, the patient we have been following, finally reached the decision point — what treatment would be best for him?

CASE STUDY

When he first heard about UPPP, he thought it had some appeal: a relatively simple operation that might eliminate his snoring, and maybe his sleep apnea, for good. However, his sleep specialist explained that he did not appear to be a very good candidate for UPPP.

Mr. Kennedy has a short jaw, so most of his obstructive sleep apnea probably arises from low in his throat. It probably would not be resolved by UPPP. In that light, the pain and risks of surgery didn't seem worthwhile.

With the advice of his sleep specialist, Mr. Kennedy decided on CPAP combined with weight loss.

At the time this book is being revised for the third edition, Mr. Kennedy has been on CPAP for 13 years. He lost 20 pounds and is at his ideal weight. He exercises several times a week and feels better than he has ever felt in his life.

Mr. Kennedy travels a lot and takes his CPAP with him in a carry-on bag. Security people in airports often ask to look in the bag, but he has never been seriously hassled about it. He recently met an airport security guard who uses CPAP himself.

He has had occasional minor problems — colds, skin irritations, poorly fitting masks, equipment breakdown. But, like the pioneers that they are, Mr. Kennedy and other CPAP users learn to solve each problem as it arises.

Mr. Kennedy feels so much better now that he has never been seriously tempted to give up CPAP. He admits that he would rather not believe that he will have to use CPAP for the rest of his life. He was only 47 years old when he was diagnosed with sleep apnea, and he still thinks of himself as fairly young and vigorous. Sometimes he feels sorry for himself that he is saddled with this weird medical machine. But . . . CPAP does work.

He did briefly try an oral appliance, but an overnight monitor showed that he was still having apneas and a low blood oxygen level with the oral appliance in place. These results rule out an oral appliance and also suggest that maxillofacial surgery is unlikely to be effective. Under the circumstances, Mr. Kennedy is not willing to trade the simplicity and effectiveness of CPAP for the risks, discomforts, and unpredictable results of surgery. Maybe some better treatment for sleep apnea will come along someday. Meanwhile he will stick with CPAP.

summary

- The best treatment is the most conservative treatment that will succeed for *you.*

- Treatments for central apnea:
  Medication
  Breathing devices such as mechanical ventilators and diaphragmatic pacemakers

- Treatments for obstructive sleep apnea and mixed apnea:
  Weight loss
  Breathing devices such as CPAP
  Oral devices such as tongue or jaw retainers
  Medication
  Surgery

- Before agreeing to surgery:
  Ask a qualified sleep specialist to estimate the chances that surgery will eliminate your sleep apnea.
  Get a second opinion from an ENT surgeon who is experienced and skilled in the surgical treatment of sleep apnea.

chapter 8

Obesity and Sleep Apnea

Simple Obesity and Obstructive Sleep Apnea

Obesity is defined as being 20 percent heavier than your ideal weight as a result of excess body fat. Not everyone with sleep apnea is obese, and not everyone who is obese has sleep apnea. However, there is a strong correlation between the two.

The Sinking Spiral

The reasons obesity and sleep apnea tend to go hand in hand are threefold:

1. In obesity fatty deposits accumulate within the layers of tissue in the neck. This causes constriction of the airway.

2. In obese people excess fatty tissue in the abdomen causes abnormal loading that interferes with the normal breathing mechanisms.

3. A sinking spiral develops, involving reduced activity and increased weight. As sleep apnea worsens, excessive daytime sleepiness (EDS) also worsens. The person becomes less active, uses less energy, gains more weight, and further aggravates the apnea.

The key to treatment is to break the cycle. Weight loss alone can effectively do this for some people. However, weight loss may be difficult or impossible to achieve as long as the sleep apnea is untreated.

CASE STUDY

Mrs. Baker had gained 50 pounds and felt increasingly exhausted. Her sleep was restless and unrefreshing, and her terrible, irregular snoring concerned her husband because she appeared to be gasping for air. Her doctor told her to lose weight and refused to refer her to a sleep center because "that's what they will tell you to do anyway."

Mrs. Baker joined a weight loss program and lost 50 pounds after spending $3,000. Her snoring improved a great deal, but it did not go away; and although her exhaustion had largely disappeared, she still felt drowsy when sitting, reading, or relaxing. Within seven months her excess weight had returned, and with it her symptoms.

Another physician agreed to refer her to a sleep center. Moderately severe sleep apnea was diagnosed. Mrs. Baker was placed on CPAP, which eliminated her sleep apnea. On CPAP and with the help of a dietitian, she again lost the weight. Now at her ideal weight, she was again studied at the sleep center. To her dismay, she still had 50 percent of her sleep apnea unless she slept with CPAP.

Looking back, Mrs. Baker realized that after her initial and expensive weight loss, her apnea had continued to leave her fatigued and had decreased her activity level. As a result, her weight had increased; as she saw herself failing, she became depressed and ate more.

Now, using CPAP, Mrs. Baker is able to maintain her new weight.

CPAP eliminates the obstructive apnea, allowing more restful sleep and a better blood oxygen level, which boost the person's energy level. The increase in energy and activity can then contribute to the weight loss effort.

*T*he Pickwickian Syndrome

The *Pickwickian syndrome* is a special type of sleep apnea that is associated with being overweight. Essentially it is severe sleep apnea combined with obesity and a chronically decreased breathing pattern called hypoventilation. This syndrome is found in approximately 5 percent of sleep apnea patients.[1]

CASE STUDY

Mr. Roberts is a 45-year-old computer programmer and former college track star. He had always been active and energetic, with many outside interests.

Mr. Roberts first became aware that something was wrong with him in 1979. He realized that he felt tired a lot of the time. He had no energy. He became less and less active, and he started to gain weight. He began to take frequent naps. Eventually he began falling asleep at work. Fortunately, his boss liked and respected him, and he was sympathetic, although puzzled. He wondered if Mr. Roberts had a problem with alcohol or drugs and hoped that in time he would be able to work it out.

Between 1979 and 1985, Mr. Roberts changed from a trim, fun-loving, lively man into an overweight, lethargic, crabby near-invalid. He was asleep, or half asleep, nearly all the time. He also had developed heart problems. His doctor was stumped.

Mrs. Roberts was desperately worried. One day she heard by chance about a new sleep disorder center and talked her reluctant husband into making an appointment.

The sleep specialist immediately recognized Mr. Roberts's problem as a variety of sleep apnea. From the information in Chapter 1, you may recognize in Mr. Roberts one of the most common symptoms of sleep apnea — excessive daytime sleepiness.

Some clues from Mr. Roberts's past might have tipped you off further — his ability to fall asleep anywhere in any position and his loud snoring. When he was in the service, he was legendary; his snoring was so horrendous that his buddies often had to carry him outside in the middle of the night so that they could get some sleep. Many a morning Mr. Roberts woke up on his cot in the middle of the parade ground.

By the time he visited a sleep clinic, Mr. Roberts was showing all the symptoms of the Pickwickian syndrome.

For centuries observers have linked obesity, breathing disorders, and drowsiness. Dionysius, the tyrant of Heracleia during the time of Alexander the Great, was described by historians as extremely obese and continually sleepy and was said to have had difficulty breathing. In fact, he is reported to have been "choked by his own fat." Magas, king of Cyrene, also was obese and was said to have "choked himself to death" in 258 B.C.

In 1816 William Wadd, surgeon to King George III of England, connected obesity, lethargy, and breathing difficulty. He described three patients who were "suffocated by fat." In 1889 another medical man, A. Morison, reported a case of an obese, drowsy man whose drowsiness improved after he lost weight.[2,3]

It was not until the 1950s that anyone came close to explaining what causes the Pickwickian syndrome. A respiratory physiologist was the first to suggest a cause-and-effect link between obesity and breathing difficulty. He proposed that obesity places an extra load on the respiratory system and suggested that this leads to lethargy and sleepiness,[2] but he failed to connect sleep apnea with the total picture. Finally, in 1965, Gastaut demonstrated the relationship between sleep apnea and excessive daytime sleepiness.

The term *Pickwickian* was first used as a medical term in an article by Bramwell in 1910. One of his patient's symptoms reminded him of the description and behavior of the fat boy, Joe, in Dickens's *The Posthumous Papers of the Pickwick Club* (1837). In Dickens's words:

> A most violent and startling knocking was heard at the door; it was . . . a constant and uninterrupted succession of the loudest single raps, as if the knocker were endowed with the perpetual motion, or the person outside had forgotten to leave off.

> Mr. Lowton hurried to the door . . . . The object that presented itself to the eyes of the astonished clerk was a boy — a wonderfully fat boy — . . . standing upright on the mat, with his eyes closed as if in sleep. He had never seen such a fat boy, . . . and this, coupled with the utter calmness and repose of his appearance, so very different from what was reasonably to have been expected of the inflicter of such knocks, smote him with wonder.

> "What's the matter?" inquired the clerk.

> The extraordinary boy replied not a word; but he nodded once, and seemed, to the clerk's imagination, to snore feebly.

> "Where do you come from?" inquired the clerk.

> The boy made no sign. He breathed heavily, but in all other respects was motionless.

> The clerk repeated the question thrice, and receiving no answer, prepared to shut the door, when the boy suddenly opened his eyes, winked several times, sneezed once, and raised his hand as if to repeat the knocking. Finding the door open, he stared about him with astonishment, and at length fixed his eyes on Mr. Lowton's face.

> "What the devil do you knock in that way for?" inquired the clerk, angrily.

"Which way?" said the boy, in a slow, sleepy voice.

"Why, like forty hackney-coachmen," replied the clerk.

"Because master said I wasn't to leave off knocking till they opened the door, for fear I should go to sleep," said the boy.

To anyone who has no experience with the Pickwickian syndrome, this scene may seem far-fetched. But Dickens was a keen observer of humankind and clearly depicted the most obvious symptoms:

- Marked obesity
- Daytime drowsiness
- Tendency to fall asleep during routine activities
- Snoring

Other features of the Pickwickian syndrome that are less obvious to the casual observer are:

- Sleep apnea
- Bluish tone to face (cyanosis)
- Abnormal breathing reflexes
- Enlargement of right side of the heart
- Heart failure

What Causes the Pickwickian Syndrome?

The Pickwickian syndrome is the result of several conditions coming together at once: sleep apnea, an abnormal breathing pattern, obesity, and usually some obstructive lung disease.[1] Some people have a breathing reflex that is not very sensitive and allows the waste gas, carbon dioxide, to accumulate in their blood (see Chapter 3). This tendency becomes worse if the person's breathing is very shallow. Obesity causes shallow breathing by interfering with the work of the breathing muscles.[4,5] This abnormally shallow breathing pattern becomes even worse when the person is lying down, and this in turn leads to frequent awakenings, sleep apnea, daytime sleepiness, low energy, additional weight gain, and so forth. A vicious circle develops, which is called the obesity-hypoventilation syndrome, or the Pickwickian syndrome. The Pickwickian syndrome may begin in childhood, and it can occur in adults who formerly were quite thin.

What Are the Effects of the Pickwickian Syndrome?

The Pickwickian syndrome leads to the same problems that result from other kinds of sleep apnea. A Pickwickian person has fragmented sleep. Deep sleep and REM sleep are reduced, sometimes nearly to zero. And because he does not take in sufficient oxygen during the night, he suffers from a kind of slow asphyxiation.[4,6]

Excessive drowsiness during the daytime is common. Pickwickian people have a remarkable tendency to fall asleep whenever there is a moment's relaxation. They often fall asleep at their desks at work, in the middle of a conversation, or while driving a car.

Mr. Roberts tells of habitually driving to work and falling asleep in the parking lot. His coworkers would come out and find him, turn off the car, and guide him in to his office, where he would spend the day sleeping at his desk. A Pickwickian doctor reported dozing off while examining a patient. He awoke to find his head resting on the patient's shoulder. A Pickwickian business executive finally sought treatment after falling asleep during a weekly poker game — he had drawn a full house (aces over kings) but then dropped off to sleep and missed the play.[7]

Serious heart disease is closely associated with the Pickwickian syndrome.[4,6,7] In addition to the risks of hypertension, stroke, and coronary artery disease that accompany obesity, there are the risks of heart enlargement, arrhythmias, pulmonary complications, and heart failure that can result from sleep apnea. There is a relatively high rate of sudden death among the obese.[6] The Pickwickian syndrome should be treated seriously because in the long term it certainly is life-threatening.

Treating the Pickwickian Syndrome

CPAP combined with weight loss is the most conservative treatment. If CPAP is not able to eliminate the sleep apnea and low blood oxygen level, a temporary tracheostomy may be used (see Chapter 7).

The medical literature is mixed in its reports about the effectiveness of weight loss in reducing the symptoms of this syndrome. However, it may be that the more weight lost, the more likely it is that the person's apnea will improve. For any particular individual there may be a critical weight above which the breathing difficulties of the Pickwickian syndrome appear. Below that, weight improvement can be expected.[7]

The combination of CPAP (to eliminate the apnea, oxygen deprivation, and debilitating daytime drowsiness) and a serious long-term weight loss program can have dramatic results. Mr. Roberts is a good example.

CASE STUDY

(continued). Mr. Roberts was put on CPAP and a weight loss program. A year after beginning treatment for sleep apnea, Mr. Roberts was quite literally a different person. He had lost 100 pounds and was full of energy. He continued to steadily lose weight and was working at regaining his health. Thanks to a sympathetic boss, he still had his job. He was also remodeling his house (doing much of the work himself) and restoring several classic cars. He didn't have time to take naps.

Some Pickwickian people treated in this way appear to have a complete "remission." They can stop using CPAP, and they appear to be cured of sleep apnea.[8]

Weight loss surgery (gastric bypass) is reported to be effective in treating the Pickwickian syndrome, reducing sleep apnea to near zero and restoring deep sleep and REM sleep.[6] However, gastric bypass surgery is not a trivial operation, and it should not be considered a conservative treatment option (see Chapter 7 for further information on treatment of sleep apnea).

summary

- Obesity is common among obstructive apnea patients.
- The Pickwickian syndrome is a form of sleep apnea caused by a combination of obesity and a shallow, abnormally insensitive breathing mechanism.
- Symptoms of the Pickwickian syndrome include:
  Obesity
  Daytime drowsiness
  Falling asleep during routine activities
  Snoring and sleep apnea
- Treatment includes CPAP and weight loss.

chapter 9

Sudden Infant Death Syndrome and Sleep Apnea in Infants

*I*s Sleep Apnea the Cause of Some Cases of Sudden Infant Death Syndrome?

Is sleep apnea the cause of *sudden infant death syndrome* (SIDS)? Probably in some cases, but the answer depends a lot on how SIDS is defined. SIDS is considered a sleep disorder, but its exact cause (or causes) remains unknown and somewhat controversial.

One authority has compared SIDS to a table littered with jigsaw puzzle pieces. "Our task is to fit [the pieces] together and to identify how many pieces are missing. One difficulty is that we don't know how many different jigsaw puzzles the pieces belong to."[1]

Current opinion is that SIDS and sleep apnea are completely separate jigsaw puzzles. In other words, some infants die from SIDS and some infants die from apnea, but they may not be dying for the same reasons.

Although SIDS probably has several causes that remain unidentified, recent evidence suggests that a significant proportion of infant deaths during sleep are due to sleep apnea.[2–4] The peak in infant sleep apnea occurs two to four months after birth, which coincides exactly with the peak in SIDS.[4]

Sleep Apnea in Infants

Variations in breathing during sleep are common — even normal — in infants. As explained by one authority, in infants "pauses in breathing are an integral part of normal respiratory behavior, are strongly influenced by age and sleep state, and do not of themselves constitute an abnormality."[5]

Normal, full-term infants are born with immature breathing reflexes. Apnea during sleep is fairly common shortly after birth, and it decreases with age as the breathing reflexes mature. Frequent or prolonged apnea events are not normal and may be a sign of a breathing problem that should be called to the attention of a doctor.

Premature infants' breathing reflexes are very immature, and these infants have more and longer apnea events than full-term infants.[6] Apnea in premature infants is normally not considered a problem unless the apnea events appear to be prolonged. However, it is very difficult to predict which premature infants will have serious apneas during their first months at home. Some pediatric sleep and breathing specialists recommend that all premature infants be sent home with an apnea monitor (described below)[7,8] or have a polysomnographic sleep study to help identify potential sleep/breathing problems.[9]

Experts disagree as to how much apnea should be considered a danger sign. Two or more apnea events of more than 20 seconds during an eight-hour period would be considered prolonged apnea.[5] Infants who show this kind of apnea during their first month of life should be considered at higher risk and need to be carefully watched.

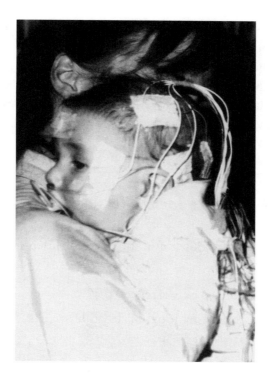

Figure 9.1
A child who is suspected of having a sleep disorder is prepared for a sleep test at a sleep center.

A*pparent Life-Threatening Events*

When an infant is found not breathing and blue, the situation is referred to as an "apparent life-threatening event" (ALTE). These infants may also be labeled "near-miss SIDS."

Doctors sometimes can pinpoint the breathing failure that causes an ALTE. Many factors can cause breathing problems in infants, including congenital heart or lung abnormalities, structural abnormalities of the face or upper airway, bacterial or viral infections, abnormal metabolism, sedatives, seizures, and gastroesophageal reflux (regurgitation of stomach contents).[10]

When an infant's apnea does not seem to be related to any of these causes, the diagnosis is simply "apnea of infancy."

A polygraphic sleep test can help diagnose the cause unexplained apnea of infancy or ALTEs.

R*isk Factors for SIDS*

The following groups of infants are considered to have a higher risk of SIDS:

1. Infants who have experienced ALTEs

2. Infants experiencing long, observable apneas (lasting more than 20 seconds)

3. Premature infants who still have apneas when they are taken home

4. Infants with a family history of SIDS

5. Infants sleeping on their stomach; soft bedding; fluffy objects in the crib

6. Smoking in the home (second-hand smoke)

Other factors include male sex and feeding practices. Male infants have a slightly higher chance of SIDS. Breast-feeding decreases the risk of SIDS.[12]

However, the "high-risk" groups of infants account for only a small portion of SIDS victims.[10,11] In the majority of SIDS cases, no previous risk factors were noted.[11]

If you have an infant you think may fall into a higher risk category, you may want to talk to your pediatrician about your concern and ask for a consultation with a sleep specialist.

*P*reventing Sudden Infant Death Syndrome

1. The most important preventive measure is to always *put a baby to sleep on its side or back,* never on its stomach. This violates a long-standing practice of putting an infant to bed on its stomach. Nevertheless, data show that on-the-back sleeping decreases the risk of SIDS. Since 1992, when the American Academy of Pediatrics made this recommendation, there has been a 38 percent decrease in the incidence of SIDS.[13] Although this is not absolute proof of the cause of SIDS, it does suggest a strong relationship between the on-the-stomach (supine) sleep position and SIDS.

2. Parents should *remove fluffy toys and bedding* (for example, sheepskin) from the crib. A baby can suffocate if its face becomes buried in these objects.

3. *Second-hand smoke* from adults smoking in the home is also strongly correlated with SIDS. Make your baby's home a smoke-free environment.

4. Every adult who cares for your infant should *know cardiopulmonary resuscitation (CPR)*.

5. *Talk with a pediatric sleep specialist* if you think your baby may be at risk for SIDS. The sleep specialist may prescribe CPAP, which has been shown to be effective in preventing infant sleep apnea.[14]

*A*pnea Monitors: Coping with Risk

A number of electronic apnea monitors are available for use at home. However, they are not foolproof.

An apnea monitor consists of sensors that are either placed under the baby's mattress or attached to the baby's abdomen. If breathing stops for a selected period of time, usually 20 seconds, the monitor signals the parents by ringing a bell and flashing a light. However, the monitors can be fooled into giving false-positive alarms, sometimes as often as 25 percent to 50 percent of the time. A lot of false alarms can be discouraging for the parents and may tempt them to turn off the monitor.[15]

The fact that monitors can also give a false-negative response is a more serious problem. That is, they may fail to indicate that breathing has stopped, when it has. This can happen if the baby stops breathing, but the heartbeat, which becomes stronger when breathing stops, is still felt by the monitor. Additionally, in obstructive apnea, when breathing stops but abdominal muscle movements are still being made against the obstruction, the monitor may misinterpret these movements as breathing. In either case the alarm might not go off until all motion has stopped, by which time brain damage or death may have occurred.[15]

Despite these drawbacks, there are cases in which a monitor might be helpful: for a premature infant who seems susceptible to prolonged apnea events; for an ALTE or "near-miss" infant whose pediatrician has ruled out other known causes of infant apnea; and for some siblings of SIDS victims who are considered to be at high risk and whose parents need reassurance.[15]

The monitor should be used for as long as the physician and parents think it is necessary. This may be from three to five months, until the child reaches an age the physician regards as safely beyond the risk of SIDS. Or the physician may wait until the child passes through an adequate alarm-free period and appears able to tolerate immunizations and respiratory infections without breathing difficulty.[10]

If an apnea monitor is to be used, the baby should be examined by a physician who is familiar with these devices in order to decide on the best type of monitor to use. In addition, a 24-hour support service should be arranged, through the doctor or the hospital, in case of equipment breakdown.

Finally, it is extremely important that everyone who cares for the infant (parents, grandparents, other relatives, babysitters) **must** be trained in CPR. If you have not had CPR training, ask your doctor to arrange it for you or ask your local Red Cross for a schedule of their classes.

Treating Infant Sleep Apnea

Most infant apnea disappears as the infant matures. SIDS is uncommon after age six months. If apnea continues beyond six months, various treatment options, including nasal CPAP, may be suggested by a sleep specialist (Figure 9.2).[3,14]

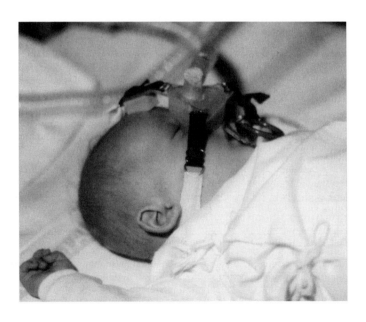

Figure 9.2
A six-week-old infant being treated with CPAP, wearing a ResCare Bubble Mask™.

*L*ong-Term Risks of Sleep Apnea

Treating infant sleep apnea is important not only to protect the infant but also in the long term. Untreated infant sleep apnea is believed to increase the likelihood of obstructive sleep apnea in adulthood. Abnormal infant breathing can cause changes in the structure and development of the lower jaw and airway. These changes, in turn, can result in the appearance of obstructive sleep apnea in puberty.[3] Therefore, it is doubly important to discuss your concerns about childhood sleep-disordered breathing with a sleep specialist.

summary

- To help prevent SIDS: put an infant to sleep on its back or side; remove fluffy bedding and toys from the crib; do not allow smoking in the home.

- Sleep apnea can result in infant death but may be the cause of many cases of sudden infant death syndrome (SIDS).

- Infants who are premature and still have apneas at the time they are sent home, who have had an ALTE or have been diagnosed as having "apnea of infancy," or who are younger siblings of SIDS infants are considered to have a higher risk of SIDS.

- Infants who stop breathing during sleep or whose breathing during sleep is noisy should receive a thorough evaluation, including a sleep study.

- An apnea monitor may be indicated for high-risk infants.

- Treatment of sleep apnea depends on the cause of the sleep apnea, as discussed in the chapter.

- Treatment of childhood sleep apnea may help avoid the development of sleep apnea as an adult.

- Consult a sleep specialist if you suspect sleep apnea in an infant.

Sleep Apnea in Older Children and Adolescents

Sleep apnea in older children is probably more common today than it was a generation ago. This is because tonsillectomies are much less common now, so many more children today have enlarged tonsils and adenoids. Enlarged tonsils or adenoids are the main causes of sleep apnea in children, but tonsillectomy and adenoidectomy are ineffective in curing 30 percent of children.[1]

CASE STUDY

Jody was a 10-year-old girl who had been snoring terribly for three years. She also made snorting noises in her sleep. She was tired and short-tempered during the day, both at home and at school. Her tonsils were large, but her pediatrician did not believe in taking out tonsils unless they were regularly becoming infected. He told the family she would outgrow this.

The family physician suggested an evaluation at a sleep center. The sleep test revealed that Jody had severe apnea, with 40 apnea events per hour. She had a tonsillectomy, her symptoms disappeared, and her temper and school grades improved markedly.

Causes of Sleep Apnea in Children

The causes of sleep apnea in children are similar to the causes of apnea in adults:

- Central apnea, the result of an abnormal breathing drive in the brain.

- Obstructive apnea, the result of a narrow or blocked airway. Airway blockage can arise from nasal obstruction resulting from a deviated septum or from allergies, large tonsils or adenoids, large soft palate, small lower jaw, and other structural features of the mouth, jaw, or throat that result in a narrow upper airway. Obesity also is a contributing factor.

- Mixed apnea, a combination of central and obstructive apnea.

Symptoms of Sleep Apnea in Children

Snoring is the most obvious symptom of childhood sleep apnea. Heavy snoring, accompanied by loud snorting, alternating with silence, is a sign of fairly severe obstructive apnea. Even lighter snoring alternating with heavy breathing may be a sign of sleep apnea that, in a child, is serious enough to need treatment.

Restless sleep and unusual sleep positions are other possible signs of sleep apnea. A child who is having trouble breathing often will thrash about, sit up, or kneel and bend forward in a position that helps to keep his airway open.

The behavioral symptoms of sleep apnea in children often are quite different from those seen in adults. Do not assume that a child with a sleep disorder must appear sleepy!

Sleepy children may actually become "wound-up," hyperactive, or aggressive. In fact, children have been diagnosed with attention-deficit hyperactivity disorder (ADHD) when their primary problem was sleep apnea or another sleep disorder. Improved behavior on Ritalin does not prove that the child has ADHD, since a child with a sleep disorder will also behave better on Ritalin. Furthermore, many children with ADHD also have sleep disorders, the treatment of which may result in improved behavior. A child who is hyperactive and who snores or has restless sleep should be evaluated by a sleep specialist to determine whether he or she has sleep apnea or another sleep disorder that needs to be treated.

Some children with sleep apnea may simply appear quiet, withdrawn, or pathologically shy. Their "good" behavior may not be perceived as a sign of a problem, even by their family.

Children whose apnea arises primarily from obesity are most likely to have the signs you would expect in an adult — daytime sleepiness and lethargy.[1]

Poor performance at school — poor concentration, underachievement, behavioral problems — is one of the most typical signs of sleep apnea. It is estimated that two-thirds of the children who are eventually diagnosed as having sleep apnea are not identified until their parents are alerted to a problem by school authorities.

Other possible signs of sleep apnea are bed-wetting, morning headache, and cardiovascular problems, such as high blood pressure and arrhythmias (heartbeat abnormalities).[2,3]

Untreated sleep apnea in children is likely to become worse and in time leads to the same kinds of cardiovascular and respiratory complications that are seen in adults. It should be considered life-threatening in the long term. Furthermore, it is impossible to overstate the disadvantages these children may suffer as a result of poor performance in school. The consequences of poor concentration and behavioral problems can affect a child for the rest of his life, so no time should be lost in treating sleep apnea.

If your pediatrician or family physician is not familiar with sleep apnea, he may fail to recognize its signs. You might want to make a tape recording of the sounds of your child's snoring and ask your doctor to refer you to a sleep specialist. It is important that a child who is suspected of having sleep apnea be thoroughly tested by a sleep specialist and that treatment be scheduled as soon as possible.

*T*esting for Sleep Apnea in Children

As with adults, diagnosis of sleep apnea and other sleep disorders (see Chapter 6) is most effectively done in an accredited sleep center. Children are more difficult to diagnose and can easily be misdiagnosed by inexperienced doctors or by sleep labs that do not have the necessary laboratory technology. The following cases show that inadequate testing can easily lead to misdiagnosis and inappropriate treatment.

CASE STUDY

Billy was 10 years old, and his teacher reported that he was having trouble paying attention in school. He was crabby and was a restless sleeper. No medical problems were identified other than allergies, which caused nasal breathing and enlarged tonsils. Billy's parents insisted on testing for a sleep disorder, and a limited test for breathing during sleep was done in their home. The results were negative and "proved" that there was no sleep problem. Unconvinced, the parents took Billy to an accredited sleep center, where a comprehensive sleep study showed mild apnea and upper airway resistance syndrome that had been missed with the simple home test.

CASE STUDY

Becky was 8 years old and had been waking up yelling and rhythmically shaking her legs. She was tired and appeared confused the next day. This happened a few times a month and was very disturbing to her parents. They took her to a neurologist, but nothing was found. She then was studied at a sleep center and was found to have a seizure disorder. Her parents agreed to start her on medications, and her episodes stopped entirely.

CASE STUDY

Mary was 7 years old and had been waking up moaning, with her legs rigid and shaking. She appeared confused, and her parents thought she looked as if she were having seizures. Her neurologic evaluation was negative, but she had some "abnormalities" in her electroencephalogram (EEG). She was diagnosed as having seizures and was given medications. She developed a severe rash. Her parents eventually took her to a sleep center, where she was diagnosed as having a night terror disorder that mimicked seizures. She was treated with counseling, and her spells gradually disappeared.

Diagnostic testing for sleep apnea in children should include a thorough physical examination, with special emphasis on the anatomy of the face, neck, and upper airway. This may include a fiberoptic examination of the airway.

An X-ray–type image of the child's head may also be needed. This can by done using several techniques, each of which has drawbacks. X-ray examinations (roentgenograms) and fluoroscopic examinations will expose the child's head to ionizing radiation, which poses a significantly greater hazard for children than for adults. Computerized tomography (CAT scan, especially fast CT) is less hazardous, and magnetic resonance imaging (MRI) is harmless, but both of these procedures are more expensive. Consult your doctor about which of these options is most appropriate.

An overnight sleep test should be performed to confirm the presence of sleep apnea, to measure the severity of the disorder, and to rule out other disorders. A multiple sleep latency test (MSLT) also should be done to measure the degree of sleepiness.

The results of a child's sleep test may be evaluated a little differently from those of an adult. Very little is known about how much apnea occurs in normal children, so it is difficult to know how much apnea should be considered "abnormal." An apnea index greater than 5 apneas per hour of sleep is considered a sign of sleep apnea in adults. Some sleep experts believe that a respiratory disturbance index (RDI, apneas plus hypopneas) of 5 is high for a child.[4]

Because adults and children with sleep apnea differ in both symptoms and sleep test results, it would be wise to look for a sleep specialist who is experienced with pediatric sleep disorders.

---

*T*reating Obstructive Sleep Apnea in Children

Because most obstructive apnea in children arises from enlarged tonsils and adenoids, the most frequent treatment is simply to remove them. The operation has some risk but is fairly routine. *However, at least 30 percent of children who have tonsillectomy and adenoidectomy will still have sleep apnea and need further treatment.*

Several other types of surgery have been used to treat sleep apnea in adults. These surgeries usually are not appropriate in a child. Because the child's bones and soft tissues are still growing, there is a chance that the obstructive apnea may disappear as growth occurs.

Medications are sometimes used in adults. The drugs used in adults either are generally inappropriate for children or have not been found to be very effective.

Continuous positive airway pressure (CPAP) is becoming the treatment of choice for children whose obstructive sleep apnea is not or cannot be resolved by tonsillectomy. Children with an abnormally small jaw structure may be placed on CPAP until they are old enough (teenaged) for surgery to be effective. CPAP is most successful in young children when the child is able to understand how the mask and equipment work and when the parents are cooperative.[5] CPAP is well tolerated by teenagers.

Weight loss usually is helpful if obesity is part of the problem. Weight loss works best if the whole family is involved in a program of weight loss and counseling.[1] Extremely severe apnea may require corrective surgery, such as uvulopalatopharyngoplasty (UPPP) or mandibular surgery, as described in Chapter 7.

Regardless of treatment, a follow-up sleep study is a good idea to confirm that the therapy has been effective.

summary

- Sleep apnea in older children usually results either from enlarged tonsils or adenoids or from obesity.

- Consult a sleep specialist if you suspect sleep apnea in a child. The diagnosis can be tricky because symptoms of sleep apnea in children may not appear to be related to sleep.

- Treatment depends on the cause of the sleep apnea, as discussed in this chapter.

- Tonsillectomy and adenoidectomy can be effective, but 30 percent of children will still have apnea and need further treatment. Insist on a postsurgical assessment of your child's breathing.

- Long-term follow-up should include periodic parental observation to be sure symptoms do not return.

chapter 11

Sleep Apnea and the Senior Citizen

*S*leep in Older People

We often assume that it is normal for older people to get less sleep during the night than younger people. This assumption often is further explained by the assumption that "older people don't need as much sleep." In fact, both of these assumptions are open to question.

It is true that people over 50 years of age typically do get less than seven hours of sleep during the night, compared with eight hours for people 19 to 30 years old. This is partly because older people awaken more often during the night and partly because they usually wake up earlier in the morning.[1] However, older people also appear to take more frequent daytime naps than young people, so an older person's total amount of sleep during a 24-hour period may be very close to the eight hours obtained by a younger person.[2]

However, the *quality* of sleep that older people get is not as good as it is in younger people. From reading Chapter 3 you know that the quality of the sleep is diminished when a night's sleep is broken up by wakefulness. Older people's sleep is lighter and more fragmented by periods of wakefulness than is the sleep of younger people (Figure 11.1).

Older people experience less deep sleep (Figure 11.2). They get almost as much REM sleep as younger people, but it is less intense.[1]

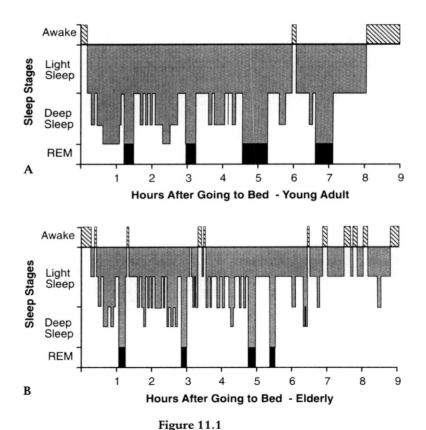

Figure 11.1
Typical patterns of sleep during one night for (A) a young adult and for (B) an elderly person. The young adult has more deep sleep and longer REM periods. The older person has more shallow, broken sleep and shorter REM periods.

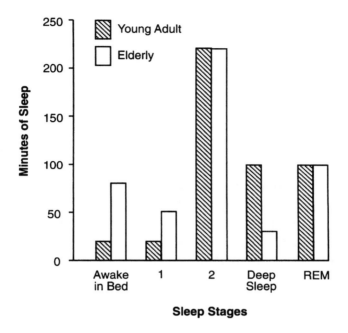

Figure 11.2

Comparison of the amount of time young people and older people spend in each stage of sleep.

Older people may be attempting to compensate for sleep lost during the night by napping. In some individuals naps may make up for the amount of sleep lost, but they do not make up for the loss of sleep quality at night. In fact, in some people naps may simply compound the problem, both by making the person less sleepy at night and by confusing the person's internal clock.

The significance of these differences between the sleep of older people and younger people is not understood. No one knows exactly why we need deep sleep and REM sleep, so the meaning of the decrease in these stages of sleep with age remains to be discovered.

*M*yths About Sleep and Aging

The majority of older people are healthy and have few, if any, complaints about sleep disturbances. Even though their sleep may be more fragmented than it was when they were younger, they do not appear to be unduly bothered by it. However, some older people do have serious sleep problems. Unfortunately, they may be discouraged from seeking help by certain myths about sleep and aging.

- Feeling sleepy is not "just part of getting old." Do not accept this explanation by family physicians, or even your own rationalizations that tell you that being sleepy during the day is "just part of being old." If you are drowsy to the point that it affects your ability to drive alertly for at least an hour, to read for 30 minutes or more, or to sit and socialize with family, the odds are that you may have a treatable sleep disorder.

- Disturbed or poor sleep is not normal. Do not accept explanations that claim that disturbed or poor nighttime sleep is "normal." Although most elderly people agree that their sleep is not what it used to be, most do not believe that poor sleep is significantly interfering with how they feel or function.

If you think your quality of life is being diminished by sleeping difficulties, do not hesitate to seek help and do not be discouraged by those who would make light of your complaints.

*R*easons for Disturbed Sleep in Older People

Sleep Apnea

Sleep apnea is one of several medical conditions that can seriously interfere with the sleep of older people. Sleep apnea has been reported in as many as 30 percent of the healthy elderly adults who have been studied.[2,3] It probably results from the gradual loss of tone in the muscles in the upper airway that occurs with increasing age.

The sleep apnea seen in healthy older people is usually very mild or moderate. In many cases it is not severe enough, or is barely severe enough, to qualify as clinical sleep apnea (i.e., more than five apnea events of 10 seconds or more during an hour, or a total of 30 or more apnea events during a night).[4]

The consensus seems to be that a mild degree of apnea in otherwise healthy older people does not normally call for treatment, provided they feel well rested. However, a suspicion of sleep apnea should not be ignored. Drowsiness and loss of mental alertness are the worst enemies of the healthy senior citizen, whose goal should be to remain as active and alert as possible. Apnea episodes contribute both to fragmentation of sleep and to a decrease in the oxygen content in the blood, which can lead to daytime drowsiness and loss of alertness. Seniors with other kinds of sleep disturbances, such as restless legs, show less daytime drowsiness.[2] This suggests that sleep apnea may be a particularly significant cause of the daytime drowsiness seen in seniors.

If you are an older person who suspects that apnea is significantly disturbing your sleep and is causing drowsiness during the daytime, you may want to contact a sleep center for an interview and potential testing. If your snoring is disturbing your spouse or partner, but you are otherwise sleeping well and have a minimal amount of apnea, Somnoplasty™ may be effective (see Chapter 7).

Leg Movements During Sleep

Approximately 40 percent of older adults experience involuntary leg movements associated with sleep. In restless legs syndrome, a person has an uncomfortable or achy feeling and an urge to move the legs. This may interfere with falling asleep. Periodic leg movements (nocturnal myoclonus) are kicking motions that occur repeatedly during sleep. These may awaken the sleeper, but often they do not and are more disruptive to the bedmate. If you or your bedmate experience either of these disorders, talk with a sleep specialist about possible treatment.

Medical Problems and Depression

Some less healthy older adults are bothered by medical problems that affect sleep (e.g., pain from arthritis, respiratory problems, frequent urination, or leg cramps).

Depression is another condition that can affect sleep. The symptoms of depression often are attributed to "just getting old" — insomnia; pessimism; loss of interest; decreased energy; poor self-esteem; poor sexual functioning; increase in health complaints, such as constipation, back pain, abdominal pain, headache; social withdrawal; decreased appetite; and weight loss.

However, it is *not* true that aging inevitably leads to these difficulties. Healthy older adults who are not depressed do not routinely experience these symptoms. If depression is the cause of symptoms such as poor sleep, it is the depression that needs to be treated, not simply the symptoms.

The treatment of medical problems and depression that interfere with sleep is best carried out in consultation with a sleep specialist, as explained later, because some treatments can further interfere with sleep.

Getting a Good Night's Sleep

The most common sleep complaint among healthy older people is that they awaken numerous times during the night.[1] People sometimes become worried about this pattern, and the worry itself — that they're "not getting a good night's sleep" — keeps them awake.

If you are a senior who is somewhat bothered by frequent awakenings during the night and drowsiness during the day, and you doubt that you have a serious sleep disorder, here are some helpful things that you can do for yourself.

1.   Practice good "sleep hygiene." That is, try arranging your daytime life so that you promote good sleep:

    a.   Eat regular meals.

b. Get more exercise every day (but don't exercise right before bedtime).

c. Go outside for a while every morning. Your biological clock needs light signals to regulate your sleep-wake cycle everyday. Indoor light is not bright enough to work very well. Morning light, even on a cloudy day, can reset your sleep-wake rhythm and help you get better sleep.

d. Eliminate daytime naps. They often are more the result of boredom than sleepiness. Find something active to do instead of napping.

e. Plan evening activities — with friends or by yourself, either outside or in the home. Look forward to a full evening.

f. Limit your caffeine intake (coffee, tea, cocoa, cola) and use alcohol moderately (alcohol actually interferes with sleep).

g. Limit your fluid intake after 7 p.m. so that you will have less need to urinate during the night.

h. Make yourself get out of bed and get dressed at a specific early hour every morning (say, 6:30 or 7 a.m.).

i. Learn relaxation techniques to relieve the tension or worries that may be keeping you awake.

2. Reassure yourself that brief nighttime awakenings are normal and that you probably are actually getting enough sleep. This knowledge alone may release you from worrying about getting a good night's sleep. That, in turn, will probably let you sleep better.

3. If these suggestions are not effective, strongly consider seeking help.

If you try these suggestions in a disciplined way for several weeks and decide they are not helpful, make an appointment to discuss the problems with your doctor. If the symptoms are not resolved, ask your doctor about a referral to a sleep clinic.

If you have a medical problem that seems to be interfering with your sleep, check with a sleep specialist for ideas about a solution that will help you sleep better.

Sometimes the treatment for one medical problem may conflict with the treatment for another. For example, some drugs taken for heart problems can make sleep apnea worse. "Sleeping pills" nearly always make sleep apnea worse, as does alcohol. Barbiturates and some antidepressants have side effects that can affect sleep. A sleep specialist is likely to know more about these effects on sleep than your family doctor does, and the two of them should work together to find the most appropriate way of improving your night's sleep.

If sleep apnea is a moderate to serious problem or if you have other conditions, such as arrhythmias (irregular heart rhythms), congestive heart failure, or respiratory problems, that are aggravated by sleep apnea, the sleep specialist may recommend treatment for your apnea. The type of treatment will depend on the kind of apnea and the severity of the problem (see Chapter 7 for treatment of sleep apnea).

summary

- Older people often get as much total sleep in 24 hours as young people do.

- However, the sleep of older people may be of poorer quality; that is, broken up by periods of wakefulness.

- Factors that can interfere with older people's sleep include sleep apnea, leg movement syndromes, pain, respiratory problems, frequent urination, medications, and depression.

- Seek help if you are persistently drowsy or if sleep disturbance is decreasing your quality of life.

- If you suspect sleep apnea, go to an accredited sleep center for an interview and possible testing.

- Mild sleep problems often can be solved by a program of good "sleep hygiene," as discussed in this chapter.

chapter 12

Finding a
Sleep Specialist

*T*he State of the Art

If your car needs new brakes, you don't take it to a windshield shop. The same is true of sleep apnea.

Find an expert.

This is especially important because sleep disorders medicine is a fairly new medical specialty, and few doctors are trained in the field. A survey of medical schools found that the average amount of time spent teaching about sleep was 20 minutes.

Because of managed care and financial arrangements with insurance companies, your doctor may want to send you to someone in his referral group who is not board certified in sleep medicine or does not even practice sleep medicine full time. Find out if your health plan is "capitated" — this means that every time your doctor orders a test it costs the clinic money. In a capitated setting you are more likely to be denied care or to be offered potentially unproven or lower quality services. The doctor often may not consciously be trying to "save" money but may have been too ready to believe claims that some service is "cheaper" and "just as good." This may sometimes be true, but do you want to be the exception?

Most established specialties, such as pediatrics, obstetrics/gynecology, otolaryngology (ear, nose, and throat), psychiatry, and so on, have their own departments in hospitals and medical schools. Medical students are taught by specialists in these fields, and they learn routines for diagnosis and treatment of illnesses in those areas. After medical school, doctors can spend several years in residency programs perfecting their skills in their chosen specialties. But very few medical schools offer courses or programs in sleep disorders medicine. Consequently, very few doctors are trained to recognize and treat sleep disorders.

In the absence of established departments of sleep medicine in hospitals and medical schools, a number of professional organizations have taken on the role of setting the standards for professionalism in the field. The American Academy of Sleep Medicine (AASM), whose members are accredited sleep centers and sleep specialists, has established the standards for the evaluation and treatment of sleep disorders. Its parent organization is the Association of Professional Sleep Societies (APSS), which also includes the Sleep Research Society (SRS). The APSS coordinates the publication of journals that deal with sleep and sponsors conferences on the latest research and treatments for sleep disorders.

Today these professional organizations are the backbone of sleep disorders medicine and the main source of learning and information exchange for professionals in the field. This will change in time. The field is growing very rapidly. The AASM hopes the major medical schools will have programs on sleep disorders within a few years. However, until systematic sleep medicine training becomes part of the medical school curriculum, the public will have to look carefully to find a qualified sleep specialist.

Q*ualifications of a Sleep Specialist*

Because so few training programs have existed, most of today's sleep specialists have done their residencies in other related specialties. In 1991 the AASM reported the specialties of their members as follows: psychiatrists, neurologists, psychologists (48 percent), pulmonologists (38 percent), and other specialties (14 percent).

These doctors have then gone on to study sleep physiology through additional fellowship programs, graduate courses, or periods of practice at one of the major sleep disorders centers. In 1993 only eight such AASM-accredited fellowship programs in sleep disorders medicine existed. They were located at Stanford University; Georgetown University Hospital in Washington, DC; Mt. Sinai Medical Center in Miami Beach; VA Medical Center in Allen Park, Michigan; Henry Ford Hospital in Detroit; University Hospital at Stony Brook, New York; the Medical College of Pennsylvania; and Crozer-Chester Medical Center in Upland, Pennsylvania.

A physician can earn a sleep specialist credential by passing the certification examination administered by the American Board of Sleep Medicine (ABSM). He becomes a board certified sleep specialist (BCSS). (Before the recent establishment of this board, the credential for a certified sleep specialist was accredited clinical polysomnographer, or ACP.) In 1998 there were approximately 1,100 board certified sleep specialists in the United States.

Some physicians who have trained in sleep medicine do not choose to become certified. Nevertheless, they may be well informed about sleep disorders. However, as in any medical specialty, a doctor's board certificate in sleep medicine assures you, the consumer, that the doctor has received special training and is qualified to carry out sleep testing and interpret the results of the tests.

You may feel hesitant to ask a doctor about his training and qualifications, but this is especially important in a new field such as sleep disorders medicine. "Are you board certified in sleep medicine?" is a perfectly legitimate question. If the doctor appears surprised by your question, you can pleasantly remind him that it is your body he is dealing with. Or you can call the American Board of Sleep Medicine (507-287-9819) and ask whether a particular doctor is certified in sleep medicine, or find a list of accredited sleep specialists on the ABSM Web site (see Appendix).

You might also ask your sleep doctor if he is a member of the AASM. Although membership in a professional group is not mandatory, it indicates something about his involvement in the field and may suggest how well he keeps up with current sleep research.

If you are reluctant to ask a doctor these questions, call his office and ask his nurse. If she can't answer your questions, ask her to find out and call you back.

Finally, it is not advisable to embark on a treatment program for a "sleep disorder" before having undergone thorough sleep testing at an accredited sleep disorders clinic. This is particularly true if the treatment involves surgery. Read Chapters 5, 6, and 7, and seek a second opinion.

Standards for an Accredited Sleep Center

An accredited sleep center is one that has met the standards established by the AASM. As of summer 1998 there were nearly 400 accredited sleep centers and laboratories in the United States. In addition, there were thousands of nonaccredited sleep labs nationwide. No one knows the exact number of nonaccredited sleep labs, but the AASM had received more than 3,000 requests from sleep labs for information about earning accreditation.

A nonaccredited sleep lab may be good, but you have no way of knowing. Your family physician also is unlikely to be intimately familiar with the details of quality sleep medicine and may just be referring you to someone in his group. However, a very wide range of quality exists, all the way down to some "street corner" sleep labs that are not reputable. The AASM has neither the funds, the staff, nor the mandate to "police" the entire field of sleep medicine beyond its own membership.

And so far no other organization or agency is keeping an eye on the quality of sleep testing that goes on in the non–AASM-accredited labs.

As a prudent consumer, if you want some assurance of professional standards in this new field, you may want to choose one of the sleep centers accredited by the AASM.

The standards for accreditation are broken down into two categories: full-service sleep centers and specialty labs.

Full-Service Sleep Centers

The requirements for accreditation for a full-service sleep center ensure that the center is able to deal professionally with the full range of sleep disorders. Here are the primary AASM requirements for a full-service sleep center:

- It must have an AASM-accredited clinical polysomnographer (M.D. or Ph.D.) on staff to read and interpret the results of sleep recordings.

- It must have a full-time physician with expertise in sleep physiology.

- It must have trained technicians to administer the sleep tests. Sleep centers are encouraged to have at least one technician who is accredited as a registered polysomnographic technologist.

- A private room must be provided for each patient, with sound, light, and temperature control and easy communication with the attendant.

- The facilities, testing procedures, and patient care must meet standards set by the AASM.

- The sleep center must pass inspection by a two-member accreditation team every five years or it will lose its accreditation.

Specialty Labs

The standards for accreditation of a specialty lab are similar but tailored to a less extensive sleep testing role. Specialty labs usually deal primarily with pulmonary medicine (breathing disorders), and the diagnostic testing they do is mostly for sleep apnea rather than for the full range of sleep disorders.

The requirements for a specialty lab include the following:

- It must have at least one pulmonary specialist on staff.
- The staff must demonstrate knowledge of the practices and procedures of sleep disorders medicine.
- The physical surroundings, facilities, testing procedures, and patient care must meet AASM standards similar to those for a full-service sleep center.

How to Locate the Nearest Accredited Sleep Center and Sleep Specialist

The AASM will mail you a booklet listing the 300-plus accredited sleep centers in the United States. Write to the AASM at the following address. Include a large, self-addressed, stamped envelope.

American Academy of Sleep Medicine
1610 14th Street NW, Suite 300
Rochester, MN 55901-2200
(507) 287-6006
www.aasmnet.org

American Board of Sleep Medicine
(507) 287-9819
www.absm.org

W*hat to Do If You Are Denied Referral to a Qualified Sleep Specialist or Lab*

You should discuss the problem with your family doctor. If he or she is unwilling to refer you to a qualified specialist, or is actually the source of the denial, you should call your Human Resources Department, union representative, or health plan agent and learn the steps you need to take to appeal the denial. If that fails, write to your state insurance commissioner, whose office can be found by calling your state capital's government information number. All states have an individual or office that supervises insurance plans and HMOs. Because of well-publicized abuses, insurance commissioners are very interested in identifying these types of problems.

chapter 13

Choosing a CPAP and a Homecare Company

You shop around before you buy a car. You may talk to several dealers, compare makes and models, and find out which dealers provide good customer service.

When you need a continuous positive airway pressure (CPAP) machine, you should do the same. You don't need to take forever to shop around. Your health is at stake, and you should start using CPAP as soon as possible after your doctor prescribes it. But some shopping can be worthwhile. After all, you will spend more time with your CPAP than you will in your car. The features of that CPAP machine and the homecare service you receive will become important to you.

*T*wo Choices to Make

You will need to select the homecare company that will sell you the CPAP, and you will need to choose a CPAP machine and its attachments. Start by asking questions at your sleep center.

1.   About homecare providers (these companies sell CPAPs and other medical equipment).

■   Ask your sleep center for a list of CPAP suppliers and homecare companies in your area, and ask whether the sleep center's medical center provides the equipment.

■   Ask your sleep center which homecare companies they recommend. Why?

■   Ask if any local homecare companies have an unfavorable reputation.

■   Ask if the sleep center can put you in touch with other CPAP users. Go to an AWAKE meeting (for sleep apnea support groups; see Chapter 15 and the Appendix) and find out which homecare companies have given good service to other CPAP users. You may find that some local branches of a particular homecare company provide better service than others. Perhaps Company A has the best service in the north end of town, but Company B has the best CPAP man on the south side.

2.   About CPAPs.

■   Which CPAP s does your sleep center think you should consider? Why?

■   Which features do they suggest you look for (mask fit, size and shape of unit, durability, adaptability, appearance, and so on)?

■ What will your insurance pay for? Call your insurance agent and ask him. This is important.

(continued). When Mr. Kennedy's sleep specialist prescribed a CPAP machine, Mr. Kennedy had no idea where to begin. His sleep center recommended that he call a homecare company. He had never heard of homecare companies. He didn't know that he could have chosen between several homecare companies in his area and that different homecare companies may carry different makes and models of CPAP. He didn't know that the features of CPAP units vary from one manufacturer to another or that he had an option of renting or buying a CPAP.

He called the homecare company that his sleep center recommended and bought the first CPAP he saw. Fortunately, he was content with both decisions. However, if he had it to do over, Mr. Kennedy thinks he would start by renting a CPAP unit. Then he would ask questions about other CPAP models and compare prices and services among several homecare companies. (Many insurance providers now prefer rental for a month or two.) He might try out several masks and CPAP models on a rental basis and decide which features were most important to him before buying his own CPAP.

Choosing a Homecare Company

If you have never dealt with a homecare company, you may not even be aware of their existence. Homecare companies (sometimes called durable medical equipment, or DME, providers) rent, sell, and service health care equipment for use at home, including mechanical ventilators, oxygen, CPAP systems, and other home health care supplies.

You can ask your sleep center representative for a list of local homecare companies, or you can find them listed in your Yellow Pages under

Medical Equipment or Hospital Equipment and Supplies. The nation-wide homecare companies have branch offices throughout the country, but not all of them may serve your area.

Questions to Ask When Choosing a Homecare Provider

Select several homecare providers and then visit their offices. See what they have to offer. Ask lots of questions. Take notes. Then compare.

1. What brands and models of CPAP do you supply?
    (A homecare company may deal with only one or two CPAP manufacturers.)
2. What are your prices for CPAP units?
3. What are your prices for parts, especially masks, tubing, and filters?
4. Can you rent a CPAP with the option to purchase?
5. How many CPAP setups do you do in a month?
6. Is the person who is going to set up my CPAP a licensed respiratory therapist (as required in some states)?
7. Do you have a selection of different masks that I may try?
    (If the answer is no, find another homecare provider right away!)
8. What services do you include in the price of a CPAP?

Here is the *ideal* service that you should receive from your homecare company:

Your first CPAP unit should be delivered to you in your home by a representative of the homecare company you choose. If you choose the sleep center, they should provide the equipment before you leave the test facility.

The representative should be trained and able to set up your system properly, making sure the CPAP is set for the pressure prescribed by your sleep specialist. He or she should instruct you about the use and care of the equipment and answer any questions you have.

The homecare representative should fit you with a CPAP mask under sleeping conditions — while you are reclining, and with the CPAP turned on. He or she should have an assortment of sizes and brands of mask available for you to try and should fit you with a mask that is comfortable on your face and does not leak. He or she should continue to work closely with you for as many days or weeks as it takes for you to feel you have a comfortable, trouble-free CPAP setup.

You should have 24-hour service in case of CPAP breakdown or emergency and the use of a "loaner" if you would be without your CPAP. Orders for new masks, filters, and other replacement parts probably will be mailed to you and should reach you within two or three days.

You should have your CPAP serviced annually. You may have to ask for this, and you may have to pay the cost of renting a replacement while your own unit is being serviced.

In reality, many homecare providers' service falls short of this ideal. You may have to go to their office to pick up your CPAP and be fitted for a mask. Some homecare companies deliver the equipment to your home, but the delivery person may not be trained to set up a CPAP (although many states now require that respiratory devices such as CPAP be applied by a licensed medical person (e.g., licensed respiratory therapist, R.N., M.D.). Some homecare providers won't let you try on a variety of masks, claiming that would be unsanitary. This is cheap nonsense and a clear signal to immediately find another homecare provider. Proper mask fitting is the most important CPAP service a homecare provider should offer. Demand it!

You can always change companies if it turns out that you are unhappy with your homecare company. Like a consumer buying a car or a dishwasher, you will need CPAP parts and service from time to time, and someday you will buy a replacement machine. A smart homecare provider should understand that you are free to take your business elsewhere and should be sensitive to your needs.

If your health care is provided by a health maintenance organization (HMO), it may have a contract with a particular homecare provider that you will have to deal with. If that homecare company won the contract by being the lowest bidder, service may be slim to none. Some homecare providers even mail CPAPs to their HMO patients — sight unseen! HMO patients may have to be very assertive to get the service they deserve. You should report in writing any dissatisfaction with the performance of a homecare company to your sleep center and to the medical director of your HMO and continue to complain until you get the help you need or are permitted to use an alternative homecare provider.

Choosing a CPAP

As with homecare companies, be prepared to ask questions and make comparisons. Keep in mind the following:

1. You need a prescription to obtain a CPAP unit from a home-care company. The prescription will tell what CPAP pressure you need and whether you need a special type of CPAP.

2. Find out what CPAP costs your insurance will cover. Most insurance companies will not cover the cost of rental or purchase of a CPAP system unless a sleep study has been done to document the medical necessity for CPAP. Most insurance companies will pay only for the standard, "bare-bones" type of CPAP unless the sleep specialist specifically prescribes and documents the medical need for a more expensive machine, such as a bi-level, variable, or "smart-PAP."

3. Consider renting for a month or two with an option to buy. Most insurance companies will pay for one month's rental.

Numerous makes and models of CPAP are available (see examples in the photos in Chapter 7). CPAP technology is growing and changing so rapidly that we cannot describe specific makes or models (the information would be out of date by the time you read this book). The important thing is to compare features. This is why it may be a good idea to rent and try out a model or two before you purchase. Each model has unique features, so the choice may seem confusing at first.

CPAP masks are sold separately from the CPAP unit. Numerous brands and sizes of masks are available (see photos in Chapter 7), and most masks can be used with most CPAP units.

The comfort and fit of the mask is so important that the next chapter is devoted to mask fit and comfort.

Let's look at three major areas of comparison among CPAP units: quality, price, and special features.

CPAP Quality = Reliability and Performance

You need a CPAP unit with:

1. Reliability. It must work properly all night, every night.
2. Performance. It must be capable of delivering a constant level of air pressure even when there is a leak around the mask.

In deciding on a brand, the least risky choice would be one of the top manufacturers. All have established track records for supplying high-quality products, parts, service, and support for their products. At the time of this writing, there are four leading manufacturers of CPAP equipment (see the Appendix for address, phone number, and web site):

- Nellcor Puritan Bennett (a unit of Mallinckrodt, Inc.)
- ResMed Corp.
- Respironics, Inc.
- Sunrise Medical (DeVilbiss CPAP products)

ResMed grew out of Baxter Healthcare, Inc., which in 1986 supported the commercial development of the original CPAP technology invented by Dr. Colin Sullivan in Australia. ResMed was the first manufacturer to incorporate several innovative features into CPAP — the universal power supply (1988); the delay timer, or "ramp" function (1989); and the Bubble Mask™ (1991).

Respironics was the first manufacturer to make CPAP units commercially available. They have steadily improved and expanded their product lines while continuing to provide good service. As mentioned in Chapter 7, the company introduced a system in 1990 called BiPAP®, with two variable-pressure settings, and have been leaders in the development of the "smart-PAP."

Healthdyne, another reliable CPAP manufacturer, merged with Respironics in 1998. Respironics has said they will continue to support existing Healthdyne products.

Nellcor Puritan Bennett has a long track record of manufacturing hospital equipment and has fine CPAP units on the market. Puritan Bennett developed a small alternative mask called the ADAM circuit, or nasal pillows, which is popular with many CPAP users.

All these CPAP manufacturers have regional or local representatives who visit the sleep centers and the homecare companies that carry their brand and train the employees in the proper use and maintenance of the equipment.

The staff of your sleep center has extensive experience with a variety of CPAP units. They may have several models that you can examine. You may want to ask them which manufacturer they prefer. Sleep centers usually choose manufacturers that they consider reliable suppliers of equipment and parts. Their choice may be a good recommendation.

Price

At the time of this writing, CPAP rentals are approximately $200 per month, and the purchase price for a basic CPAP is about $1,200. You probably will have to purchase the mask and tubing separately (about $150 total) (these prices may vary across the country). The mask material tends to absorb oil from the skin and to become stiff, needing to be replaced about every six months, so that is a recurring expense. Some CPAP models have nonwashable air filters that need periodic replacement.

More complicated CPAP-type machines are more expensive. Bi-level units rent for about $250 per month and cost about $2,600. "Smart" CPAPs rent for about $250 per month and sell for around $1,800.

Compare the prices for a particular model among several local homecare companies. Ask what additional equipment and services they provide for that price. Find out what costs your insurance company will cover.

Special Features

Each make and model of CPAP has features that make it unique. Your particular lifestyle, taste, or leisure activities may make one model more appealing to you than another.

CPAP masks and mask fit. This topic is so important that we have devoted a whole chapter to it. Please read Chapter 14.

CPAP sound. Are you or your bedmate sensitive to noise during sleep? Listen to the sound of several CPAPs *under normal operating conditions*, that is, while the CPAP is turned on, set at your prescribed pressure, and someone is wearing the mask and breathing normally. (It will sound different if it is turned on at a lower or higher pressure or is not being worn by someone.) Most CPAPs are so quiet that they produce only a gentle "white noise," which some people find actually lulls them to sleep. Listen to both the sound of the machine and the escaping air.

Ramp or not? Many CPAPs have a "ramp" feature, which starts the machine at a low air pressure and increases it slowly over a period of 5 to 45 minutes. Many people find that this gradual increase in air pressure allows them to go to sleep more easily, especially when they are first getting used to CPAP. The ramp feature sometimes can be part of the CPAP prescription. If you want to be able to use a ramp, ask your sleep specialist to specify a ramp in the prescription.

CPAP size and shape might be important to you. Does the CPAP unit need to fit on your nightstand, or can it just sit on the floor? If you travel a lot, will it be easy to carry?

CPAP appearance. Is the appearance of the CPAP important to you? Do you care what it looks like sitting on your bedside table? Some models look more like medical devices, whereas others blend more naturally into the bedroom setting.

Humidifiers. Some people find that their nasal passages become stuffy or dry when using CPAP. A humidifier can help alleviate these problems. Some CPAP models have a built-in humidifier; some humidifiers heat the water, whereas others do not. If you experience nasal stuffiness or dryness on CPAP, you may want to ask your sleep specialist about a humidifier. The drawback to using a humidifier is the need for strict cleanliness; you must wash a humidifier daily to prevent mold growth. The other drawback is cost, which can be $100 to $400 depending on whether it is heated. Insurance companies usually will pay for a humidifier only if the doctor prescribes one.

Present and future lifestyle. You may want to give some thought to future activities — things you would enjoy doing once you have more energy. It is common for CPAP users to discover that soon they are able to be more active than they had been when they were slowed down by sleepiness or poor health. What would you like to do when you feel better? Take a trip to Europe? Invite your sweetie to spend the night? Go car camping, backpacking, or traveling across the country in a recreational vehicle (RV)? Charter a sailboat . . . ? What features of a CPAP would enable you to fulfill that wish? If you are a car camper or boater or if you have an RV, what electric source will you want to use, and how easily can your CPAP be adapted? Many active CPAP users are looking forward to the advent of more battery-friendly models. One avid backpacker is lobbying for a mini-CPAP machine that could run on solar batteries attached to his hat! Who can even imagine the wonders that technology may bring?

Traveling with CPAP

1. By all means, *do* take your CPAP with you when you travel. Don't ruin your vacation or business trip with groggy days and sleepless nights.

2. Your CPAP should *always* be in your carry-on luggage. Do not check a CPAP through as baggage — the risk of loss or damage is too high. Most CPAPs will fit into a carry-on bag and slide easily under an airplane seat. The slimmest new

models even fit in a briefcase. Some manufacturers offer an attractive carrying case that probably is roomy enough to also hold a woman's nightgown and cosmetics.

3. Durability. Select a CPAP that has a durable case if you plan to travel with it.

4. Electrical adaptability. U.S. electrical circuits operate at 110 volts and 60 Hz (cycles per second). Many European countries use 220 to 240 volts and 50 Hz. If you travel outside the United States, find out which CPAP models can be plugged into or readily adapted for European circuits. Luggage shops and travel catalogs sell a set of adapter plugs that will connect your CPAP to any plug in the world. If you often take long airplane flights, you may want to inquire about which CPAPs are approved for use on an airplane (110 V, 400 Hz).

5. Manufacturer's information. This can be useful at airport security (although CPAPs hardly ever are questioned anymore), customs, or in case of an equipment failure or emergency. Carry a manufacturer's brochure that describes your CPAP and includes phone numbers of people to contact in case of emergency. If you plan to travel in a foreign country, ask the manufacturer to send you a foreign language brochure and a company contact in that country.

6. CPAP travel accessory kit. Frequent travelers advise carrying the following, just in case: a three-prong plug, a six-foot extension cord, an extra fuse, an extra of any small connectors between mask and tubing that might get lost or damaged, and adhesive or duct tape.

Do-It-Yourself CPAP and "Self-Titration"

An unfortunate trend in CPAP treatment is the "take it home and try it out" school of medical practice. Some people who are suspected of having sleep apnea — sometimes without even the simplest of sleep tests —

are being handed CPAP machines and told to "just give it a try." What is wrong with this practice?

1. Do-it-yourself CPAP is trial-and-error medicine. The doctor is handing over his responsibility as diagnostician and healer to the patient, creating an unfair burden and usually an impossible task.

2. Do-it-yourself CPAP does not determine whether the patient has sleep apnea, another sleep disorder, or a medical condition that will remain untreated.

3. Do-it-yourself CPAP is unlikely to adequately treat the patient even if he does have sleep apnea. The patient has no idea what pressure to use. The pressure setting for CPAP should be custom-set ("titrated") for each patient in order to properly treat the sleep apnea without overtreating it. If a "self-titrated" patient is actually able to use the CPAP and actually does feel better, he still may not be adequately treated and his sleep apnea may continue to worsen.

4. There are hazards in both undertreatment and overtreatment with CPAP. Too low a pressure can leave the patient with sleep apnea symptoms that can result in the long-term effects of sleep apnea — high blood pressure, increased risk of stroke, heart attack, or heart failure. Too high a pressure can lead to poor acceptance of CPAP, poor sleep, increased mask fit problems, increased nasal problems, and in some severe cases cardiopulmonary problems.

5. Do-it-yourself CPAP is a waste of money. It does not give the patient the support he needs to use CPAP regularly and successfully. Most do-it-yourself CPAP patients will remain untreated because the CPAP will stay in the patient's closet.

One reason we are seeing do-it-yourself CPAP is the increased pressure on HMOs and other medical providers to save money by treating patients as efficiently and inexpensively as possible, but this clearly is a short-sighted and false economy. If the patient remains improperly diagnosed and untreated, the long-term costs of untreated sleep apnea — automobile accidents, stroke, heart attack, heart failure — predictably are going to be much higher than if the patient had a sleep study and was properly titrated on CPAP in the first place.

What About "Smart" CPAP?

Another reason for do-it-yourself CPAP is the advent of "smarter" CPAPs. Smart CPAPs are the latest development in CPAP technology. Smart CPAPs are supposed to be able to detect the patient's changing breathing patterns during the night and adjust the pressure to the patient's needs.

There is a misconception that anyone can send a patient home with a smart CPAP and diagnose and treat sleep apnea. In reality, smart CPAP is still under development and should be considered somewhat experimental. Most smart CPAPs have not been studied long enough to evaluate their capabilities and weaknesses. For example, each manufacturer has a different method of determining how much pressure to use and when to change pressure. As a result, the comfort for the user varies considerably from one manufacturer to another, and some systems simply seem to work better for some patients than for others.

Initially the smart CPAPs have been useful mainly in the sleep lab to aid in diagnosis of sleep apnea and to determine the appropriate CPAP pressure setting for a patient. The smart CPAP's computer stores data about the patient's breathing and the pressures used during the night, and those data can be downloaded to help the sleep specialist diagnose and prescribe treatment pressure for the patient.

Sometime soon smart CPAP will be appropriate for at least some patients to take home for the night and return to the sleep lab for a diagnosis and a prescription for treatment. However, that time has not quite arrived yet.

Smart CPAPs should be used under the direction of an experienced sleep specialist who is not simply trying to save money but actually knows that it would be highly effective in your particular case.

- Ask your sleep center for a list of homecare providers and CPAPs to consider.

- Ask your insurance agent which CPAP costs it will cover (purchase, rental, parts, service).

- Consider renting a CPAP while you shop for a homecare company and the CPAP model of your choice.

- When choosing a homecare company, compare local reputation, the brands of CPAP they sell, prices, and services.

- When choosing a CPAP, consider quality, price, recommendations from a sleep center, and unique features, such as size, shape, durability, adaptability, appearance, sound, and availability of ramp setting and humidifier.

- If someone hands you a CPAP and tells you to go home and try it, run and find yourself a sleep specialist.

chapter 14

The CPAP Mask: Getting Fit

*I*t's your first night at home with your CPAP. It's time to go to bed. You're a little anxious about this new equipment in your bedroom.

You're also kind of excited and hopeful. That morning in the sleep lab, after your first night of CPAP, you woke up feeling pretty good! If you can sleep like that every night, you'll be a new person!

Getting Started: 10 Steps

Who can remember everything the CPAP technician said about using this equipment? Because it's all so new, it is a good idea to get ready for that first night on CPAP sometime during the day, when you're not tired. Then at bedtime, when you do feel tired and may not have a lot of patience left, everything will go more smoothly.

Here are 10 steps to a good night's CPAP.

1. Wash your face very well to remove all the skin oils. This will help the mask seal nicely against your skin and it will be less likely to leak. It also will make the mask last longer. (Of course, you will wash the mask every morning as soon as you get up, so those skin oils don't sit on it all day.)

2. Arrange the tubing so it will lie or hang comfortably and not tug on your mask or fall off the bed. Some suggestions are to bring it up over the headboard; attach a fat rubber band to a cup hook in the wall above the bed and loop the tubing through the rubber band; bring the tubing under the blanket from the foot of the bed (this warms up the air a little). Many people use two lengths of tubing for more flexibility.

3. Hook up the tubing to the CPAP, which can sit on the floor, on a table, or even in the closet if there is plenty of air circulation.

4. Turn on the CPAP at full pressure. (Don't use the "ramp" until you have finished adjusting the fit of the mask at full pressure.)

5. Attach the tubing to the mask, and put on the headgear and mask.

6. Pull the mask out from your face and hold it there. Then inhale while you lower the mask to your face.

7. Lie down in bed.

8. If the headgear needs adjustment, adjust it while you are lying down. If your headgear has been adjusted for you by your CPAP technician, it may not need adjustment now. If the mask starts leaking, first try pulling it out from your face and reseating it. If you adjust the tension on the headgear, do it a little at a time. The trick is not to get the headgear too tight, or (surprisingly) the mask may leak even more. Once you have the headgear adjusted properly, you can just

slip it off and on over your head without unfastening it each time you remove the mask.

9. If you want to use the ramp feature, activate it now. Have it "ramp" up to full pressure in about 20 minutes.

10. Now just lie there for awhile and relax. Think about the beach or the clouds or your favorite restful place. Get a good night's sleep!

*M*ask Fit and Leaks

Causes of Leaks and Chafing

Air leakage around the mask and chafing of the bridge of the nose are two of the most common problems with CPAP. The reasons usually are

1. The mask is the wrong size or shape, or

2. The headgear is too tight or unevenly adjusted.

Your CPAP mask must fit securely and comfortably. Getting the mask to fit properly is probably the biggest frustration most people encounter with CPAP. Most people find that they need to experiment with the mask for a while to get a comfortable, leak-free fit.

Your homecare provider should be willing to try different sizes and brands of mask until you have an acceptable fit. If you experience leaks, chafing, or other problems, you need to immediately ask for help from your homecare company provider. If the homecare company representative doesn't respond, complain directly to your sleep specialist.

Always try on the masks with your CPAP machine running and attached to the mask.

What steps can you take to get a leak-free fit? Tell your homecare provider that you would like to:

1. Try a smaller mask. All masks come in at least two sizes, some in as many as a dozen!

2. Try a larger mask.

3. Try several different brands of mask.

4. Try "nasal pillows," a smaller version of a mask that fits up into the nostrils. Also called an ADAM circuit. Many people prefer them.

---

*T*he Wide Variety of Masks

Mask and headgear designs are constantly changing, so anything we write here will probably be out of date by the time you read it. But here is an example of the wide variety that should be available to you through a good homecare provider. This is just a sampling, not a complete list or an endorsement of any particular product.

Respironics makes a basic mask that has been the "standard" workhorse CPAP mask. Many people have been using that style of mask for 12-plus years and wouldn't change. It comes in several variations and eight sizes. Respironics also makes a gel mask (the GoldSeal™), which is heavier but feels rather neat and seals nicely against the face. It comes in seven sizes. Their Monarch® mini-mask fits up under the nose and has been redesigned with a swivel that should make it easier to wear. Respironics also makes several different types of headgear that you might want to try. They publish a brochure that illustrates all of their masks and headgear.

ResMed makes two interesting masks. The Mirage™ is popular with many patients. It is small and light and now comes with more flexible tubing, which allows more movement. It comes in only two sizes. It is very sensitive to face oil and must be washed very well every morning. The Bubble Cushion® mask is a very soft-fitting mask. It comes in several versions and many sizes. ResMed makes a variety of headgear alternatives and a chin strap that is useful for a person whose mouth falls open during sleep.

Nellcor Puritan Bennett developed the ADAM system, also called nasal pillows, which is a great favorite with many people either for every-night use or as an alternative to the mask. Nasal pillows are small rubbery cones that fit into the nostrils (see Figure 7.3). The tricks with these are:

1. to get the right size (the cones come in six sizes), and
2. to point them into your nostrils in the right direction and at the right angle.

You can get an angle adapter to adjust the angle. (You may have to educate your homecare provider about the angle adapter — for some reason they seldom know about it.) Nellcor Puritan Bennett also makes "standard" style masks out of both vinyl and silicone, which is convenient if you have an allergy to one or the other. Finally, they have an interesting marketing brochure that pictures all their many CPAP parts and accessories.

Most masks can be worn with any CPAP machine. Exceptions: Respironics' Virtuoso machine and Aria LX machine set in alarm mode will not work with some masks. Also, some masks tend to leak at CPAP pressures above approximately 15.

Mask fit is a very individual thing. What fits one person's face and works well with his or her sleeping style may not work for another person. Listen to the suggestions of other people, but then try out the alternatives for yourself.

By testing the fit of several masks and fiddling with the adjustments, you will eventually hit on the right combination.

Experiment. Don't give up!

Other Mask-Fitting Tricks

Overtightening the headgear is a common reason for chafing on the bridge of the nose. If your mask fits properly, you shouldn't have to tighten the headgear to the point of chafing.

Spacers. Several masks have different sizes of spacers that you can stick on at the top to change the tilt of the mask. Try wearing the mask a little looser and changing the size of the spacer.

Cleanliness of both mask and skin is extremely important for discouraging leaks and skin irritation and prolonging the life of your mask. Wash your face every night before putting on the CPAP. If you have very oily skin, you may want to use a mild astringent, such as witch hazel, around the nose. The most important thing you can do to extend the life of your mask is to wash it with a mild, fragrance-free, oil-free soap as soon as you take it off in the morning. Let the mask air-dry. Drying the mask by running the CPAP with the mask on the end of the hose will dry out the mask and shorten its life.

A go-between. If you still have a leak, and you have tried different brands and sizes of mask, you might try putting a soft, cushiony material between the mask and your skin. This also works for people who are allergic to the mask material. Microfoam™ tape (from the 3M Company; ask your homecare representative) can be taped to the mask. Or you might try using a go-between, which is a shield to keep the mask from touching the skin. To make a go-between, cut a 4- or 5-inch square (a little larger than the footprint of the mask) out of soft, white fabric, such as felt or thin terrycloth, and then cut a big triangle out of the middle for your nose to fit through. Place the fabric between the mask and your face.

A worn-out mask will fit poorly, leak, and cause chafing. A silicone mask should last for 12 to 18 months, depending on the oiliness of your skin and how careful you are about cleanliness. Skin oil causes the mask material to become stiff. Order a new mask as soon as the old one starts leaking, chafing, or fitting poorly. Skin abrasions from an ill-fitting mask are difficult to heal.

Sore spots. Once you have a sore spot, healing may be difficult because the mask will tend to irritate it every night. To prevent abrasion of the bridge of the nose and/or promote healing, look for wound-care products such as Restore™ or Duoderm™. Ask your homecare representative. You also might try Second Skin™, a blister remedy that is sold in stores that sell running shoes or sports equipment. If you are using nasal pillows, you can lubricate the nose openings with a non-greasy product such as Ayr™, a soothing saline gel that can help prevent irritation, or K-Y® Jelly.

Switch-offs. Some people switch back and forth between a mask and nasal pillows every few nights. They say this helps prevent irritation in the same places every night, and it gives them some variety.

There have been rare cases of eye irritation or infection either caused or aggravated by air escaping from around a poorly fitting mask. In the event of eye irritation, notify your sleep specialist. CPAP probably will have to be discontinued until the irritation clears up.

O*ther Common Mask-Wearing Problems*

Claustrophobia and Mask Removal

Some people have trouble keeping the CPAP mask on all night. They may have a feeling of suffocation or claustrophobia, or they may unconsciously pull the mask off during sleep. This is quite common, and sometimes it is just a matter of getting used to the feeling of the mask.

If you continue to have either of these difficulties for more than a week or two, contact your sleep specialist and discuss the matter with him. This problem sometimes is the result of nasal obstructions that are interfering with the CPAP. If this is the case, your sleep specialist will want to figure out the cause of the nasal obstruction, whether it is from allergies or another structural blockage. He may suggest treatment for the nasal obstruction to make CPAP more effective and comfortable for you.

The suffocating feeling sometimes is an anxiety about having the nose covered, and there are ways to work through it so that you can reach a point of being able to sleep quietly without being bothered by CPAP.[1] Talk this over with your sleep specialist and try his suggestions.

Dry Mouth

Some people find that their mouth dries out during the night wearing CPAP. This usually results from sleeping with the mouth open. Sometimes it is because the nose is congested and the CPAP air cannot get through. Sometimes it is simply a habit. If you have dry mouth and a stuffy nose, you may want to discuss nasal obstructions with your sleep specialist. You need a working nose in order for CPAP to work well. If the open mouth is a sleeping habit, you may want to try using a chin strap to help keep your mouth closed. Keeping a glass of water by the bedside is another good idea.

Nasal Congestion, Dryness, or Runny Nose

Congestion, sneezing, dry nose, or very runny nose can be temporary responses of the lining of your nose as it becomes accustomed to the CPAP pressure. If you have these problems for more than a few weeks, you might want to talk to your sleep specialist about using a humidifier (see Chapter 13). A number of CPAP units come with a humidifier, and all can be used with a separate humidifier. A nonheated humidifier is simpler and less expensive, but it requires a warm bedroom to be very effective. A heated humidifier will work better in a cold bedroom, but it will cost more and is a little more difficult to keep clean. Ask your home-care provider which humidifiers they recommend. Your doctor probably will have to specifically to prescribe a humidifier in order for your insurance to cover the cost.

If your nasal congestion is caused by allergies, ask your sleep specialist to recommend a decongestant. Some products are better for people with sleep apnea than others.

Noise

The newer CPAPs are so much quieter than the vacuum cleaner–like earlier versions that noise almost isn't an issue anymore. If noise is a problem for you or your bedmate, there are many creative options. An obvious solution is earplugs. Try the kind that are shaped like soft, foam cylinders. They are sold in industrial safety stores and are quite comfortable. If you have had your CPAP sitting next to you on the floor or on a nightstand, try moving it to the foot of your bed. If your bedroom closet is roomy and has good air circulation, you can run your CPAP unit there. Leave the door open several inches to let in air. You can even run the CPAP from a hallway or an adjacent room if you have long enough tubing. One ingenious CPAP user bracketed the machine to the ceiling of the room below the bedroom and ran the tubing up through a hole. These are the kinds of creative solutions you will hear about at AWAKE meetings from people who have been there.

All Night, Every Night — The Importance of Compliance

People fail to use their CPAP for many reasons. The most common cause of noncompliance usually is inadequate follow-up care — the user has not been properly introduced to CPAP, he does not receive proper follow-up help, or he does not understand what sleep apnea will do to his health if he does not use his CPAP regularly.

Your Ticket to Enjoying Life

You should understand that CPAP is literally a lifesaver for you. You need to use CPAP every time you go to sleep — even for naps, even when you spend just one night away from home. Use CPAP because it offers you better health and longer life than you can expect if your sleep apnea is not treated. CPAP is your ticket to enjoying the things in life that are most important to you — instead of giving in to sleepiness, exhaustion, and poor health.

If you are having an equipment problem, your sleep center and homecare staff should help you with troubleshooting. If your sleep center does not automatically offer the degree of continuing care you need, do not hesitate to request additional attention. You should receive whatever assistance you need to continue your CPAP treatment.

The key is to ask for help, and ask again, until you get it.

What If You Still Need Help?

If you:

- Don't have a sleep specialist.
- Don't have a well-staffed sleep center to turn to.
- Don't have a good homecare provider to help you.

Then the next best thing is a support group — other people with sleep apnea. Here are some sources of support. The Appendix gives details about now to reach the following:

- AWAKE groups (local sleep apnea support groups)
- American Sleep Apnea Association
- Internet newsgroups and chat rooms (take their information with a grain of salt)
- CPAP equipment manufacturers' local representatives (buy some filters from them, then ask for advice)

Other patients, possibly contacted through an AWAKE group, can be enormously helpful because they have been through the experience and can understand what you are dealing with. There is no problem that cannot be worked out. Solve the problem so that you can continue with the treatment and get on with your life. A CPAP unit does nobody any good if it spends the night unplugged in the closet.

---

*T*reatment Effectiveness

"I feel cured. Can I stop using CPAP?" Probably not. It is very common for people to report dramatic results from treatment. In fact, they often feel more improvement than has actually occurred. After uvulopalatopharyngoplasty (UPPP) surgery, a person may feel "completely cured" only to discover after retesting that he still has 50 percent of his sleep apnea. So don't assume that your sleep apnea has necessarily been thoroughly treated just because you feel better. Most important, don't assume that you can stop treatment because you feel better. Your sleep apnea will come back if you stop treatment.

Sleep apnea patients usually are asked to return to the sleep center after a specified period of treatment to be retested to verify that the treatment is effective. This is true not only for CPAP users but also for sleep apnea patients who are being treated with medication and those who have undergone surgery.

Another reason to be retested is if your treatment has not given you as much improvement as you had expected. A patient occasionally returns for retesting and the technicians find that the pressure on his CPAP unit was not properly set. Or the sleep specialist discovers a second sleep disorder that was missed during the initial sleep test. If you think you should be feeling better than you are, contact your sleep specialist.

Periodic retesting is important for all patients to make sure that the treatment remains effective over the years and that there is no return of the symptoms of sleep apnea. Most sleep centers will tell you when they want you to return for retesting. If yours does not tell you, ask.

On Being a Pioneer

Today's sleep apnea people are medical pioneers. You are helping to teach the medical community how to recognize and treat sleep apnea. You are helping the sleep disorder centers to learn how to meet their patients' needs. You are helping the medical researchers and medical equipment manufacturers to invent better treatment methods.

The sleep disorders field is young, and it still has some weaknesses. The understanding of sleep apnea is not yet widespread throughout the medical community, but there are many well-informed doctors, many excellent sleep specialists, and many superb sleep centers in the United States and throughout the world.

Most important, today there are simple, effective treatments for

TABLE 14.1

CPAP Problems and Who to Call for Help

	SLEEP SPECIALIST	SLEEP CENTER	HOMECARE COMPANY	AWAKE GROUP
Equipment Problems				
Mask fit, other problems, day-to-day use	Solutions to medical problems: (allergy, infection, inflammation, medications)	Advice, suggestions, troubleshooting	Choice of models, sizes; advice	Advice, suggestions, troubleshooting
Breakdown, repairs			24-hour service	
New products, updates		Advice, information	New equipment	Advice, information
Compliance and Mental Adjustment				
Use/nonuse of CPAP	Discuss problems Encourage Refer for counseling	Problem solving: mask fit, skin irritation	Mask fit, mask leaks, mask size, type, humidifier, service	Encouragement, support, education, problem solving
Treatment Effectiveness				
	Schedule retest	Discuss need to retest		

sleep apnea that didn't exist even two years ago. There is hope now for many people who previously could not expect to see their sixtieth birthday.

You and your partner need to be assertive, well-informed consumers in this new field. Make sure your needs are met, because in a new field it's a little bit harder than it should be to get things done. Be patient, but not too patient. Be stubborn. Don't give up! Make sure your doctor listens to you. Seek the best-equipped, best-staffed sleep centers. Ask questions until you get answers. Learn the treatment options. Choose the conservative treatment over the risky one. Seek a second opinion on surgery. Find the experienced surgeons. Keep after your insurance company until they pay for your care. Demand service from your homecare provider or switch to a competing company. Let them know if you are dissatisfied. And demand adequate follow-up care. It's your life.

summary

- Expect to go through a temporary adjustment period as you become accustomed to using CPAP.
- Patience, persistence, trial and error, asking questions, and demanding service are the keys to solving CPAP equipment problems.

chapter 15

Follow-Up Care: Living with Sleep Apnea

*E*veryone with sleep apnea shares the hope that someday this disorder can be cured and forgotten. Unfortunately, no sure cure exists today, and treatment with CPAP remains the best alternative for most people.

Until a few years ago, people with sleep apnea had a choice between drowsiness, illness, and probable early death, or a permanent tracheostomy. Today, like butterflies from cocoons, CPAP users can emerge from their private twilight, spread their wings, recapture their health, and rekindle their lives.

Problem solved. Right? Well, no. Unfortunately, adjusting to CPAP sometimes is not quite that easy. Yet sleep apnea is a long-term proposition for most people. Treatment must be continued on a regular basis if people with sleep apnea are to stay healthy.

If we were to listen in on an AWAKE group, the magnitude of the adjustment to CPAP would be obvious from the conversation. New CPAP users invariably are concerned with basic problems: mask leaks, stuffy nose, irritated skin, and dry mouth. We also would hear proof that these problems can be solved. Experienced CPAP users' interests move on to other topics — the newest CPAP models, the latest gimmicks for camping with CPAP, and the lack of public awareness about sleep apnea.

CPAP Equipment: Troubleshooting

So you have tried CPAP and are ready begin using it at home. If you have not read Chapter 13 on choosing a CPAP unit and a homecare company and Chapter 14 on selecting and fitting a CPAP mask, you might want to do so now.

Patience and Persistence Pay

Every new CPAP user goes through a period of adjustment, becoming familiar with using the equipment, becoming accustomed to wearing the mask, sleeping with it on, and keeping it clean. As a new CPAP user, you will go through this adjustment period. Some people get used to CPAP in a few nights and never have a single problem, but most people encounter some frustrations. The most common ones are difficulty with the fit of the mask and the headgear, leakage problems, stuffy nose, and dry throat. In addition, some people take a while to get used to the sound of the motor running during the night or of air escaping through the vents.

Chapter 14 on mask fitting contains some specific solutions to these common problems.

All CPAP adjustments are temporary, but they certainly can be annoying. They require perseverance on the part of the CPAP user and his family — perseverance until the person feels comfortable enough with the CPAP equipment and enthusiastic enough about its effectiveness that he is willing to continue to use it every night.

In order to reach this level of comfort with CPAP, people with sleep apnea need good follow-up care from their health care providers. Follow-up care affects more than just health. Nearly every aspect of a person's life may be touched by the quality of the continuing care he receives — his image of himself, his family relationships, his sexual life, his vitality and enjoyment of social and leisure activities, his work performance, his career — indeed, his life expectancy.

*F*ollow-Up Care Determines Your Future Good Health

The key to effective treatment of any medical disorder is a question of compliance — does the person use the treatment and use it consistently?

Surveys have shown that the cornerstone of compliance for CPAP is follow-up care — is the person receiving the kind of support he needs to be able to follow the treatment? As one health care team has stated, "The most brilliant sleep diagnosis is meaningless if the plan for treatment is misunderstood or if the patient is non-compliant. Sleep specialists have a commitment to the patient to go beyond diagnosis."

If a person with sleep apnea is simply handed a CPAP machine and told to go home and use it, the chances of his continuing the treatment are very poor. On the other hand, in sleep centers whose follow-up care is thoughtful and thorough, more than 8 of 10 CPAP users will continue to use the equipment faithfully and successfully every night.

*G*etting the Care You Need

Let's assume your doctor has prescribed CPAP, since that is the most common treatment for sleep apnea. You probably will find that the recipe for trouble-free treatment involves two main ingredients:

1. Problem solving and perseverance with CPAP.
2. A team effort.

Your Team

You should consider the following people to be members of the team that is dedicated to helping you get on with life:

- Your spouse or partner
- Other family members
- The sleep specialist
- The sleep center staff
- The family physician (perhaps)
- The representative of the homecare company that supplies the CPAP equipment
- AWAKE, the patient support group
- You — the person being treated for sleep apnea

Friends and Family

How are friends and family involved in follow-up care? Close friends and family members are important sources of support. It is good for them to be included in the treatment process so that they can be interested and well-informed about CPAP from the beginning. If friends and family are enthusiastic about the results of the treatment and can be encouraging and tolerant during the frustrating but temporary adjustment period, the person with sleep apnea will feel happier about using CPAP on a regular basis.

Your bedmate and family may take awhile to get used to having CPAP around the house and to the notion that you need to use it when you sleep. It may help if everyone thinks of CPAP as they would a pair of eyeglasses. The first person who ever wore eyeglasses probably looked fairly peculiar, but it must have been worthwhile to see better, and people soon got used to the idea. CPAP is like a pair of eyeglasses — a device that solves a problem and enhances life. With that outlook CPAP may seem less like a weird piece of medical equipment and you may feel less like an "invalid" and more like someone who just happens to have sleep apnea.

Your team includes two important groups of professionals — sleep center staff and homecare providers. Let's look at how they can contribute to your continuing care.

*T*he Sleep Center's Role in Follow-Up Care

The Ideal Follow-Up

The sleep specialist who prescribes your sleep apnea treatment probably will emphasize the importance of sticking with the treatment. It will be up to members of the sleep center staff and the homecare company to work with you from then on, making sure you are able to carry out the prescription.

Some sleep centers have a staff member who acts as CPAP contact person; takes care of follow-up; arranges appointments with nutritionists, counselors, and other specialists; and generally makes sure that people's questions get answered and problems get solved.

The trained staff person should be available to make sure that the treatment — be it a weight loss program or a CPAP unit — is tailored to your individual needs. The staff should remain available to you and your family to answer questions and help solve any problems that may arise in the future.

The ideal solution is found at sleep centers that have an actual follow-up clinic to which all patients are referred, whether they are being treated at the sleep center or by an outside physician. The follow-up clinic offers self-help meetings for people with sleep disorders and their families; monitors the progress of treatment; refers people for nutritional counseling, supervised exercise programs, psychological counseling, and other services as needed. This type of comprehensive follow-up for sleep apnea is becoming more common as sleep centers become bet-

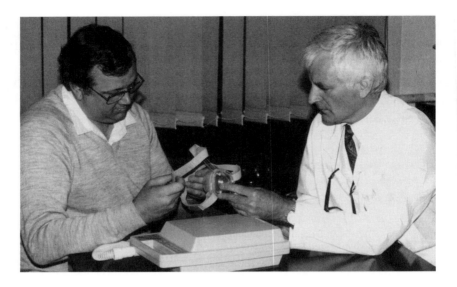

Figure 15.1
A CPAP user consults a sleep center staff member about the use of his machine.

ter established and able to provide more staff services.

Make it your business to arrange to have an annual follow-up appointment with your sleep specialist, and call immediately if you notice a decline in your ability to tolerate CPAP, if you have equipment problems, or if you notice a return of snoring, daytime sleepiness, or other sleep apnea symptoms.

*P*roblems with Sleep Centers

In some cases follow-up care is not what it should be for a number of reasons. First, sleep disorder treatment is a new field and is still in a period of rapid change. Some small sleep labs may do only sleep testing and may pass along the treatment and follow-up care to a family physician, who may have little experience with sleep apnea and little time to do adequate follow-up.

Most sleep centers are extremely busy, and some simply do not have enough staff to do complete follow-up with every patient. They are torn between the demand to diagnose new patients, including many whose health is seriously jeopardized by untreated sleep disorders, and the need to keep up with the growing backlog of people under treatment who need continuing care.

You, the patient, are caught in the middle. As always, the key is to ask for help *and to keep asking.*

If you can get in touch with an AWAKE group, the nationwide patient support network (discussed later), you may find that other people with sleep apnea can help you. They are especially resourceful in solving CPAP equipment problems.

*H*omecare Companies

What to Expect

Your homecare representative should be your chief CPAP equipment problem solver. This relationship typically begins when the homecare company representative delivers your first CPAP unit to your home (see Chapter 13 for a list of other services to expect from a homecare company).

Homecare representatives often are respiratory therapists who have been trained by the manufacturer of the CPAP equipment. They should understand the features and operation of the equipment and should make sure that the mask and headgear fit you properly.

As you begin to use your CPAP, call your homecare representative right away if you continue to have leaks around the mask, discomfort, or other difficulties. A persistently poor-fitting mask can be so discouraging that you may feel tempted to give up on CPAP altogether. Don't! Call your homecare representative before you reach that extreme. He should be available to work with you until you are happy with the results. That is the business of a homecare company, and you are paying for the service.

In case of an actual equipment breakdown, you can call your homecare company anytime, night or day. A broken CPAP results in a breathless, sleepless, stressful night and is a major inconvenience. Veteran CPAP users recall that the fan belts in the old models had a way of failing the night before a crucial meeting or during an important business trip. A good homecare company would deliver a new fan belt at 2 a.m. if a patient needed one. You should expect nothing less than prompt, dependable, 24-hour emergency service from your homecare company. If they cannot give you same-day service for repairs, they should provide a "loaner" CPAP for you to use until your unit is repaired. (Loaners may not be free unless your CPAP unit is still under warranty.)

CPAP equipment breakdowns are rare, but don't wait for one to happen. If you suspect your CPAP is developing a problem, have your homecare company check it over immediately. Also have them test the pressure once or twice a year. Some CPAP manufacturers recommend an annual maintenance checkup.

Problems with Homecare Companies

Like other service-oriented businesses, homecare companies vary in their quality and diligence. The homecare respiratory therapists who come to the home generally are sympathetic and helpful, but there seems to be a fairly high turnover rate and service may vary as a consequence. The therapist may or may not be familiar with a particular model of CPAP equipment. He may or may not know how to answer pertinent questions or solve complex problems that may arise.

In addition, communication between sleep centers and homecare companies may be incomplete. Homecare representatives typically know very little about sleep disorders or how they affect the patient. They may have never visited a sleep lab and may have no idea what a patient has experienced in undergoing a sleep test. Conversely, your sleep center may not be familiar with the capabilities, limitations, and service records of all the homecare companies in your region.

Consequently, you, the client, are the communication device that sits between the sleep center and the homecare company. You are in a position to educate the homecare people about sleep apnea and its effects on your life. If their service does not meet your needs, explain and complain. If you are dissatisfied, change companies. If your insurance does not allow you to change companies and you have received poor service, complain bitterly — in writing — to your insurer, your physician, and your state insurance commissioner.

You also can educate the sleep center about which homecare companies are doing their jobs well and which are not. Sleep centers can use this information to encourage better service and to steer other patients.

In summary, remember that when you buy or rent a CPAP from a homecare company, part of what you pay for is "service," and you should expect that service to be good. If your homecare company does not satisfy your needs, find another one.

*A*WAKE: *Your Support Group*

Other people with sleep apnea can play an enormously helpful role in your follow-up care. Some sleep centers encourage regular meetings of sleep apnea people and their families, both before and after treatment. Individuals have a chance to meet other people who have faced the same worries and solved the same problems with which they themselves are grappling. Such support groups can be extremely reassuring and resourceful.

There is a nationwide network of sleep apnea support groups called AWAKE (Alert, Well, And Keeping Energetic). AWAKE groups operate in conjunction with an existing sleep center. The clinic staff usually launches the group with the participation of a core of interested people who have sleep apnea. From then on the members operate the group, with support from the sleep clinic staff and sometimes from representatives of homecare companies. Some groups meet monthly; others, less frequently.

The purpose of AWAKE groups is to give people with sleep apnea an

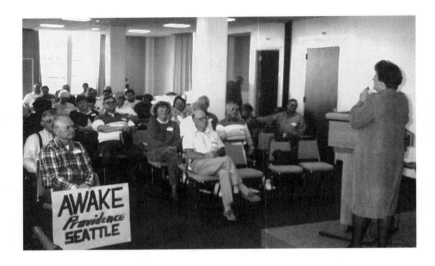

Figure 15.2
An AWAKE meeting.

opportunity for both support and learning. They share their experiences, problems, solutions, and successes, and they exchange information. Some groups publish newsletters. Many groups invite speakers to their meetings — doctors, homecare representatives, CPAP manufacturers — representatives, and so on.

By January 2000 there were over 200 AWAKE groups throughout the country, with more being started all the time.

Ask your local sleep center or homecare company representative for the location of the nearest AWAKE group, and by all means try to attend a meeting. If there is no AWAKE group near you, you may be able to help start one with the cooperation of your sleep clinic. Don't be in the position of sitting at home reinventing the wheel when you could so easily be helped by the combined experiences of dozens of other people like yourself who have found creative solutions that they are eager to share. You, in turn, will have the pleasure of helping other people by sharing your own insights and answers.

AWAKE is affiliated with another source of patient support, the American Sleep Apnea Association (ASAA), a national dues-for-membership organization for people with sleep apnea and their families and friends. This organization, which was founded in 1992, is dedicated to public education and fundraising for research on sleep apnea. Members receive an interesting quarterly newsletter. The addresses of the national AWAKE Network office and the ASAA are in the Appendix.

*M*ental Adjustments to Sleep Apnea

Mental adjustments are part of getting used to CPAP. As a new CPAP user, you will have to become accustomed to seeing yourself as someone who needs this rather unusual piece of equipment to maintain good health. Some people, particularly young people in their 40s with sleep apnea, may understandably have difficulty accepting the image of themselves as people with a chronic medical condition.

It is natural to wonder how this treatment process is going to affect relationships with friends and other members of the family. Will your children think you are an invalid? What about your sex life? Will your wife or husband still find you attractive? What will your new lover think about that CPAP on your nightstand?

CASE STUDY

Mrs. Carter worried the first time she spent the night in the home of friends. What would they think? Would the sound of the CPAP disturb the baby sleeping in the next room? On her first business trip after starting to use her CPAP, she felt self-conscious around her associates and wondered what they thought about her carrying her CPAP onto the plane.

For months Mrs. Carter scurried around feeling as if she had to conceal the fact that she had a sleep disorder and required the use of an unusual piece of medical equipment.

In time, she tentatively began to talk with friends and associates about sleep apnea and found that they were interested, curious to learn more, and very supportive. She even began to feel good about educating people and realized that she had become a kind of ambassador for sleep apnea.

"Eventually," Mrs. Carter says, "you simply reach a point of accepting yourself as a person who has sleep apnea and uses a CPAP. Period. And you get on with life."

Depression can be an unexpected but fairly common result after sleep apnea is successfully treated, and it demands effective follow-up attention.

Why would a person become depressed after successful treatment? This can happen when a person undergoes a big change in a very short time, from sleepy and sedentary to awake and active. Following successful treatment, former sleepy people may be pushed abruptly into the active life surrounding them. Friends and family may suddenly interact with them more and expect more of them, and they may doubt their own ability to perform. Family conflicts and feelings of social inadequacy may arise. The former patient may feel at a loss about how to deal with this change.

Another common reaction is one of bitterness over having lost a number of good years of one's life. Many people with sleep apnea have spent their prime midlife years in a state of deep somnolence. When they "awaken" after treatment, they feel resentment and loss at having been robbed of those good years. People may need to allow themselves time to grieve before they can let go of those years and get on with life.

Other adjustments occur in the workplace. After treatment a former sleep apnea patient often is literally a different person from the lethargic, sleepy person to whom his colleagues had become accustomed. It may take him awhile to retrain those coworkers to recognize the "new" person's capabilities. If you find yourself in this frustrating situation, it may help to remember to allow both yourself and your colleagues some time to adjust.

The spouse or partner of someone who has been treated for sleep apnea also has some adjustments to make. She has become accustomed to living with a sleepy person. Perhaps she has had to take over many of the family, household, and financial tasks and now must learn to share them again. If her spouse has been very sick, she may even have emotionally prepared herself for his death. The transformation of her partner into someone with unexpected vitality and energy may be a shock. She may not at once welcome such an abrupt change. She may be surprised to feel a confusing mixture of emotions, from anxiety to resentment to guilt.

These are all significant adjustments, and most people with sleep apnea have to deal with some of them.

This is another advantage of attending an AWAKE meeting. You will discover that you are not alone in having mental adjustments to make. It may help to talk with others who have been through similar experiences. Counseling can also be helpful, for the individual or the whole family, giving people a chance to talk over their concerns. Your sleep specialist or the sleep center staff can recommend a counselor.

You — *The Captain of Your Team*

You are the most important member of your treatment team! You are responsible for your health — for choosing, using, cleaning, and caring for your CPAP equipment. If you have unsolved treatment problems, ultimately the best solution is for you to be utterly relentless. Don't give up! Ask questions until you get answers. You can find answers if you are persistent. Reread Chapter 14 on CPAP problem solving and start trying alternatives. If you still have a problem, get in touch with the sleep specialist who first evaluated you. If he is difficult to reach or is unable to help, ask him to refer you to someone who can. Keep asking. Every problem has a solution. You can find it.

summary

- Sleep centers and homecare companies have an obligation to provide adequate follow-up care. Arrange to have an annual follow-up visit with your sleep specialist. Call immediately if you notice a drop in your ability to tolerate the device, equipment problems, or a return of your symptoms.

- If you have follow-up questions or problems, assert yourself until your needs are met, or find another sleep center or homecare company.

- AWAKE is an excellent nationwide patient support organization for people with sleep apnea. Local chapters have scheduled meetings. To locate the closest AWAKE chapter, contact your sleep center, homecare company, or call the AWAKE Network.

chapter 16

Alternative Medicine and Sleep Apnea

Mr. Chambers was having trouble getting used to his CPAP machine. He was still waking up many times during the night and still feeling fatigued during the day. His sleep center scheduled him for a trial on BiPAP™. With BiPAP he slept through the night and felt refreshed the next morning. He arranged to buy a BiPAP unit and began using it nightly.

At about the same time, Mr. Chambers read an article that promoted magnetism as a treatment for a number of medical complaints, including fatigue. The article described the miraculous cures of several patients and claimed that these anecdotes "proved" the effectiveness of magnetism. The author of the article offered several magnetic products for sale.

Mr. Chambers wanted to feel better. He was impressed by the testimonials of the patients who had tried magnetism. He ordered several hundred dollars worth of magnetic bracelets, magnetic shoe inserts, and magnets to put in his mattress and pillow.

Today Mr. Chambers feels more alert and energetic than ever before. He is convinced that magnetism has revitalized him.

A new field of medicine offers fertile ground for quackery. Unscrupulous people are quick to exploit people's hopes and fears. Claims of miracle cures for sleep apnea are already germinating among the "alternative" medical practitioners.

Who Can Diagnose Sleep Apnea?

Let's be clear on this. For an accurate diagnosis of sleep apnea, you need an overnight sleep test that follows standardized procedures. The results should be evaluated — and the treatment prescribed — by a well-trained, preferably accredited, sleep specialist.

Any alert doctor may suspect sleep apnea by looking at you, asking you if you snore, and performing a physical examination. But for an exact diagnosis and appropriate treatment, you need a sleep test.

Can "Alternative Medicine" Treat or Cure Sleep Apnea?

"Alternative medicine" cannot treat or cure sleep apnea. There is no sure cure yet for sleep apnea. There is effective treatment, but the sleep apnea will return if the treatment is stopped.

Sleep apnea is a complicated disorder, and the choice of the correct treatment depends on many factors, as explained in Chapter 7. The only known effective treatments for sleep apnea include one or more of the following:

1. CPAP
2. Weight loss for some people
3. Certain medications for some people
4. Certain surgeries for some people
5. A dental appliance for some people

*Q*uack Detection: Rules of Thumb

Quacks are experts at appealing to our natural desire for a swift cure. Like most people with sleep apnea, Mr. Chambers didn't want to sleep with a CPAP machine. He was disappointed that his initial CPAP treatment hadn't worked as well as he had expected. He wanted a simple answer. He fell prey to a quack.

How can you recognize a quack? Who can you believe? And does it really matter if, like Mr. Chambers, you seem to feel better? Yes, it does matter, for two practical reasons:

1. Quackery is expensive. If you are on a limited budget, you can ill afford to spend your income on quack remedies.
2. Quackery can kill you, either directly with a dangerous product or indirectly by failing to treat a fatal disorder properly.

If you want to avoid the expense and risks of quackery, here are some rules of thumb.

1. Be skeptical. Question anything that seems too good to be true.
2. Ask for credentials. What are the credentials of the person who is making the claims? Can he document any special training that qualifies him to dispense medical advice?

3. Follow the money. Who profits if you spend your money on this product or service? Is the cost reasonable, or is someone offering you a dime-store item for $50?

4. Question the research. This is hard to do if you are not a scientist. Good scientific research follows scientific method.

How Does Scientific Method Work in Medicine?

Scientific method dictates that a new treatment must be fairly tested. Multiple experiments, repeated in more than one laboratory, must test and retest the treatment to determine its safety and effectiveness and to measure whether it works any better than a placebo.

The placebo effect predicts that *any* treatment will automatically make you feel better. For example, a sugar pill, a pain killer, and the doctor's hand touching your aching back are all likely to ease your pain. So when humans are involved, the experiment must be double-blind, that is, neither the patient nor the experimenter must know what is being tested.

When the first data on CPAP were published by Sullivan's group in Australia in 1981,[1] the rest of the medical community was skeptical. Experiments were repeated in other laboratories around the world, and the good results were verified. CPAP has now become a treatment principle that has shown results in many thousands of cases.

Now what about the "miracle of magnetism?" Let's run that notion through our rules of thumb. Does it seem too good to be true that tiny, weak magnetic fields could abolish the effects of sleep apnea? Does the "authority" selling this theory have medical credentials? Who profits from the sale of the magnets? He does. Has he done double-blind experiments and published the results in a reputable medical journal? No.

Someone else has done the research, though. A Wisconsin sleep center measured sleep apnea symptoms with and without magnets and found "no benefit from magnetic therapy."[2]

What do you think? Is there proof that magnets revitalized Mr. Chambers? Or was his improvement more likely the result of his new BiPAP?

*A*lternative Medicine: What It Can and Cannot Do

With a few exceptions, most alternative medical practices are not harmful, provided they are not used as a substitute for good primary medical care. They may be helpful in promoting better health. At worst, they may be needlessly costly. None can offer you the cure for sleep apnea.

If you feel compelled to try alternative methods, at least be scientific about it. Discuss your ideas with your doctor, perform a controlled experiment yourself, and then be prepared to return to the sleep lab to find out whether there has been a measurable improvement in your sleep apnea.

*T*wo Very Bad Decisions

One of the worst decisions you could make would be to stop using the treatment your sleep specialist prescribed while you try some new alternative. If you want to experiment with unconventional treatments (provided they are not harmful), at least continue to use your CPAP at the same time. If you stop using CPAP, your sleep apnea is guaranteed to return, and it will become worse over time.

The second bad decision would be to use an alternative practitioner as your primary or only doctor. Most alternative practitioners have limited medical training. They may fail to diagnose a serious disease (diabetes, cancer, heart condition) that could be fatal if it is not properly treated. If you must experiment with alternatives, do so in addition to good, regular, conventional medical care.

But Maybe This Really Is the Cure!

It's true — the cure for sleep apnea may indeed exist in some obscure alternative medical treatment. Many scientific discoveries originate outside the conventional establishment. The medical establishment is very slow to accept new ideas. Unconventional treatments are viewed with skepticism bordering on suspicion, and their proponents are often ostracized by the medical community.

Sleep disorders medicine itself is a perfect example of how long it takes to integrate a new concept into mainstream medicine. Sleep disorders research has been going on for more than 40 years, but sleep disorders medicine is only now beginning to be taught in medical schools. Yet this very skepticism is what guards the public from the quacks. New medicine has to prove itself through scientific method and peer review in the medical journals. This process prevents abuse and exploitation of the public by incompetent scientists, unscrupulous industries, and personal greed.

The system is not perfect. Some bad science is reported in the medical journals. Some good treatments take longer than they should to reach the patient. Progress seems slow, but continual advances are being made, and examples of what can happen when the review process breaks down (e.g., thalidomide) show us the value of deliberate skepticism and medical conservatism.

If a sure cure for sleep apnea exists today, the medical community hasn't heard about it, much less had a chance to test it scientifically. Prudence suggests that we keep on using our CPAPs and remain patient and skeptical.

summary

- Rules of thumb for detecting medical quackery:
  Be skeptical.
  Ask for credentials.

Know who profits and whether the product or service is worth the money.
Learn whether the research followed scientific method.

- Keep using your CPAP if you decide to try alternative therapies.
- Do not use an alternative practitioner as your only or primary physician.

Addresses, Products, and Services for People with Sleep Apnea

*T*he AWAKE Network: *Sleep Apnea Support Groups*

AWAKE is the national sleep apnea patient support network. Your sleep center's CPAP coordinator should know the nearest AWAKE group. If not, you can locate the nearest AWAKE group or obtain guidelines on starting an AWAKE group by contacting the American Sleep Apnea Association (see below).

*A*merican Sleep Apnea Association (ASAA)

The American Sleep Apnea Association (ASAA) is a national membership organization for people with sleep apnea, dedicated to public education and support for medical advances in sleep apnea. Information on AWAKE support groups in your area; CPAP support;

information on legal, workplace, and other issues affecting people with sleep apnea. Individual membership: $25. Quarterly newsletter.

American Sleep Apnea Association
1424 K Street NW, Suite 302
Washington, DC 20005
Phone: 202-293-3650
FAX: 202-293-3656
http://www.sleepapnea.org
To find a local AWAKE group, e-mail awake@sleepapnea.org.

---

*A*merican Academy of Sleep Medicine (AASM)

The American Academy of Sleep Medicine (AASM) (formerly the American Sleep Disorders Association, ASDA) is the professional sleep medicine organization, comprised of individual members and accredited member sleep centers and sleep laboratories. Contact them or visit their web site for a list of accredited sleep centers.

American Academy of Sleep Medicine
1610 14th Street NW, Suite 300
Rochester, MN 55901-2200
507-287-6006
http://www.asda.org

---

*A*merican Board of Sleep Medicine (ABSM)

The American Board of Sleep Medicine (ABSM), associated with the ASDA, is the organization that tests and certifies physicians as sleep specialists. You can find out whether a particular physician is board certified in sleep disorders medicine by contacting the ABSM.

507-285-4377
http://www.absm.org

N*ational Sleep Foundation*

This nonprofit organization's mission is to improve the quality of life of people with sleep disorders and to prevent catastrophic accidents related to sleep deprivation and disorders.

The NSF publishes excellent brochures on each of the sleep disorders. Read their publication on sleep apnea on their web site. For a copy of their sleep apnea brochure, send your request and a self-addressed, stamped, business envelope to:

National Sleep Foundation
1522 K Street NW, Suite 500
Washington, D.C. 20005
http://www.sleepfoundation.org

S*leep Disorders Dental Society (SDDS)*

For a list of dentists in your region who are familiar with the use of oral appliances for treating sleep apnea, check the SDDS web site or send your request and a stamped, self-addressed business envelope to:

Sleep Disorders Dental Society
10592 Perry Highway, #220
Building 1, Suite 1204
Wexford, PA 15090-9224
724-935-0836
http://www.thesdds.org

W*ake Up America*

The Coalition to Wake Up America is a grassroots advocacy group that encourages citizen action in support of research and medical and public education on sleep disorders. To become involved, contact:

Wake Up America
701 Welch Road, Suite 2226
Palo Alto, CA 94304
650-725-6484
http://www.stanford.edu/~dement/wua.html

---

*S*leep Apnea on the Internet

Worldwide Web Pages (as of 5/00)

Medical Sleep Disorders Web Sites, operated by medical organizations, information generally reliable:

SLEEPNET

Information, many links to other sleep sites, list of accredited sleep centers, forums, other resources, from Stanford School of Sleep Medicine.
http://www.sleepnet.com

THE SLEEP WELL

List of AWAKE groups online, Wake Up America, legislative updates, much sleep disorders info, many resources.
http://www.stanford.edu/~dement

SLEEP HOME PAGES

Many links to sleep information, and resources; forum.
http://bisleep.medsch.ucla.edu

SLEEP MEDICINE HOMEPAGE

Many links to sleep information and resources.
http://www.users.cloud9.net/~thorpy

Sleep Apnea Patient-Run or Patient-Oriented Web Sites, medical information should be verified:

A.P.N.E.A.NET

News and information on sleep apnea from a patient's point of view.
http://www.apneanet.org

A.W.A.K.E. group home pages:

CHICAGO AREA AWAKE GROUPS

Contact A.P.N.E.A. NET for information.
http://www.apneanet.org

SEQUOIA SLEEP DISORDERS CENTER AWAKE GROUP, REDWOOD CITY, CA

http://www.sleepscene.com/awake.htm

SUMMIT MEDICAL CENTER, OAKLAND, CA

http://www.summitmed.com/awake.htm

INTERNET SLEEP APNEA FORUM

http://www.sleepedu.net/forums/apnea/apneainfo.html

Contacts for Other Sleep Disorders

RESTLESS LEGS/PERIODIC LIMB MOVEMENT IN SLEEP (RLS/PLMS)

http://www.rls.org

NARCOLEPSY NETWORK

http://www-med.stanford.edu/school/psychiatry/narcolepsy
e-mail: Narnet@aol.com

YOUNG AMERICANS WITH NARCOLEPSY (YAWN)

http://www.yawn.org http://www.yawn.org

Internet discussion group: **http://egroups.com/list/narcolepsy/**

CPAP Manufacturers

Below are the major manufacturers of CPAP equipment and accessories as of 1998.

- Nellcor Puritan Bennett (a unit of Mallinckrodt, Inc.)
  2800 Northwest Blvd.
  Minneapolis, MN 55441-2625
  800-497-4979

- ResMed Corp.
  10121 Carroll Canyon Rd.
  San Diego, CA 92131
  800-424-0737
  http://www.resmed.com

- Respironics, Inc.
  1501 Ardmore Blvd.
  Pittsburgh, PA 15221-4401
  800-345-6643
  http://www.respironics.com

- Sunrise Medical (DeVilbiss CPAP products)
  7477 East Dry Creek Parkway
  Longmont, CO 80503
  800-333-4000

CPAP by Mail

You probably should not get your first CPAP by mail. It is most helpful to begin your CPAP experience with a local homecare provider, where you should have an opportunity to try a variety of CPAP equipment and should expect help, information, and support in getting started on CPAP.

However, in the future, depending on your satisfaction with the prices and service for your first CPAP, you may wish to explore other sources, including other local homecare providers.

The Internet is opening up the market for CPAP supplies such as filters, masks, headgear, and even replacement CPAPs, and prices are becoming more competitive—a welcome development for CPAP users.

Admittedly, the reason for the lower mail-order prices is that you do not receive the personal mask-fitting and trouble-shooting service that you should receive from a local homecare provider. You will be "on your own" and must be prepared to sacrifice service for lower prices.

One good Internet source is listed below. You may find others. Be sure to compare prices, and consider asking for references from other customers before buying.

CONJO Distributing: CPAP equipment and supplies at 20% to 60% below retail. CPAP tips, custom headgear. Call or visit the web site for a price list.

P.O.Box 2069
Tri-Cities, WA 99302
Phone 509-735-1842
FAX 509-735-1884
http://www.cpapman.com

S*leep Position Monitor*

For information about the effectiveness of changing sleep position as a treatment for sleep apnea and for information on sleep position monitors, check the following reference:

Cartwright, R. D. Effect of Sleep Position on Sleep Apnea Severity. *Sleep* 1984; 7(2):110–114.

W*eight Loss*

Good Sources of Sensible, Well-Balanced Recipes

The Pritikin Program for Diet and Exercise, by Nathan Pritikin with Patrick M. McGrady, Bantam. Excellent low-fat, low-sugar, low-salt, low-calorie, high-fiber recipes.

Don't Eat Your Heart Out Cookbook, by Joseph C. Piscatella, Workman Publishing. Good low-fat, low-salt, low-sugar recipes, not as low-calorie as Pritikin.

General Diet Guidelines

You can turn many of your favorite recipes into low-calorie recipes by doing the following:

1. Eliminate fats and oils (butter, margarine, other shortenings, dairy, and other animal fats). To keep food from sticking while cooking, use a nonstick pan. To sauté use a little water or bouillon instead of butter or oil. Refrigerate foods overnight and skim off the congealed fat the next day. Substitute low-fat or nonfat products for products that are high in fat—nonfat milk and yogurt instead of regular; yogurt instead of sour cream; low-fat cheese such as part-skim mozzarella instead of fatty cheeses such as cheddar and jack; chicken or turkey instead of beef. Eat more seafood.

2. Cut down on sugar. Pritikin's recipes often use a small amount of frozen apple juice concentrate in place of sugar. This juice contains only a small amount of sugar and adds just the right hint of sweetness.

3. Cut down on salt. Use herbs instead.

4. Eat lots of fresh vegetables and fruits. They are bulky and fill you up, they are low in calories, and they are full of vitamins and minerals.

5. Use whole-grain products (flour, bread, rice, pasta, and so on) instead of highly refined products. Whole-grain products are bulkier, so you will feel full on fewer calories.

You can actually have fun inventing your own low-calorie versions of favorite recipes, using more healthful substitutions. Exercising your creativity in the kitchen makes dieting more enjoyable. You can design your own great weight loss recipes.

*D*rugs That Can Make Sleep Apnea Worse

Many medications can make sleep apnea worse by making you drowsy or by disturbing your sleep or breathing. Be sure to tell your sleep specialist about all of the medications you take, both over-the-counter and prescription drugs. He may want to adjust dosages or suggest alternatives.

Some common over-the-counter (nonprescription) drugs, such as antihistamines, can make sleep apnea worse. Ask your pharmacist about all nonprescription medications that you take frequently. Can they cause drowsiness, breathing problems, or insomnia? Can he suggest alternative medications with fewer side effects?

The following prescription drugs can cause problems for people with sleep apnea. (This is not a complete list.) If you are taking any of these drugs (or their generic form), or if you suspect that a medication may be affecting your sleep, be sure to discuss these matters with your sleep physician.

TABLE

Drugs That Can Cause Drowsiness or Apnea or Insomnia

The x's indicate the chances that a person taking the drug will experience the problem listed. (Based on data from *Physicians Desk Reference*, 1993)

x   = small chance (problem affects fewer than 10% of people taking the drug)

xx = moderate chance (problem affects 10% to 25% of people taking the drug)

xxx = common problem (affects more than 25% of people taking the drug)

	DROWSINESS	APNEA	INSOMNIA
Actifed with Codeine Cough Syrup	xxx		
Alfenta		x	
Alferon N			xx
Ambien	xx		
Anafranil	xxx		xx
Anaprox, Anaprox DS	x		
Anestacon	xxx		
Asendin	xx		
Atgam		xx	
Atrofen	xxx		x
Benadryl	xxx		xxx
Bentyl	x		
Buspar	xx		x
Cardura	x		
Catapres, Catapres TTS	xxx		
Centrax	x		
CHEMET	xx		
Clozaril	xxx		
Combipres	xxx		
Cylert		xxx	
Cytadren	xxx		
DHC Plus	xxx		
Dantrium	xxx		
Depo-Provera			x

	DROWSINESS	APNEA	INSOMNIA
Desyrel	xxx		x
Dilantin with Phenobarbital	xxx		
Doral	xx		
Duragesic	xx	xx	
Emcyt			x
Emete-con	xxx		
Empirin with Codeine	xxx		
Ergamisol	x		
Esgic-Plus	xxx		
Exosurf		xxx	
Fioricet	xxx		
Fiorinal	xxx		
Flexeril	xxx		
Floxin			x
Habitrol	x		x
Halcion	xx		
Hismanal	x		
Hylorel	xx		
Hytrin	x		
IFEX	xxx		
Innovar		xxx	
Intron A	x		x
Kerlone			x
Klonopin	xxx		
Limbitrol, Limbitrol DS	xxx		
Lioresal	xxx		x
Lopressor HCT	xx		
Ludiomil	xx		
Lupron			x
Lysodren	xxx		
Marinol (Dronabinol)	xx		
Marplan	xxx		
Mazicon	x		
Mepron	xx		
Minipress	x		

	DROWSINESS	APNEA	INSOMNIA
Minizide	x		
Moban	xxx		
Nalfon 200	x		
Naprosyn	x		
Nicoderm			xx
Orudis			x
Parlodel	x		
Paxil	xx		xx
PedvaxHIB	xxx		
Permax	xx		x
Phenurone	x		
Phrenilin	xxx		
ProSom	xxx		
Prostep	x		x
Prostin VR		xx	
Prozac	xx		xx
Pyridium Plus	xxx		
Reglan	xx		
Restoril	xx		
Retrovir	x		x
Ritalin			xxx
Rynatan, Rynatan-S	xxx		
Rynatuss	xxx		
Sanorex			xxx
Seconal	xxx		
Sectral			x
Sedapap	xxx		
Seldane, Seldane-D	x		xxx
Sinequan	xxx		
Soma, Soma with Codeine	xxx		
Stadol	xxx		xx
Suprane		xx	
Survanta		xxx	
Symmetrel	xx		
Synarel			x
Tavist, Tavist-1, Tavist-D	xxx		

	DROWSINESS	**APNEA**	**INSOMNIA**
Tegretol	xxx		
Temaril	xxx		
Tenex	xxx		x
Theo-X	xxx		
Toradol	x		xx
Trandate	x		
Transderm Scop	x		
Tranxene, Tranxene-SD	xxx		
Trinalin	xxx		
Tripedia	xx		
Valrelease	xxx		
Ventolin			x
Versed	xx		
Videx			xxx
Visken			xx
Wellbutrin			xx
Wytensin	xx		
Xanax	xxx		xxx
Xylocaine	xxx		
Zoladex			x
Zoloft	xx		xx

References

Chapter 1

1. Young, Terry, Mari Palta, Jerome Dempsey, James Skatrud, Steven Weber, and Safwan Badr. The occurrence of sleep-disordered breathing among middle-paged adults. *N Engl J Med* 1993; 328(17):1230–1235.
2. Dement, William. Statement on the Findings and Recommendations of the National Commission on Sleep Disorders Research, Field hearing before U.S. Senate Appropriations Committee, Portland, Oregon, November 4, 1992.

Chapter 2

1. Aldrich, Michael S. Automobile accidents in patients with sleep disorders. *Sleep* 1989; 12(6):487–494.

2. Stoohs, R., L. Bingham, A. Itoi, C. Guilleminault, and W.C. Dement. Cross-sectional study of the prevalence of OSA in a population of long-haul truck drivers. Reported at the European Sleep Research Society meeting in Helsinki, 1992.

3. AMA Council on Scientific Affairs. Report #1. American Medical Association, June 1996.

4. Young T., J. Blustein, L. Finn, and M. Palta. Sleep-disordered breathing and motor vehicle accidents in a population-based sample of employed adults. *Sleep* 1997; 20(8):608–613.

5. Partinen M., and H. Palomaki. Snoring and cerebral infarction. *Lancet* 1985; 2:1325–1326.

6. Hung J, E.G. Whitford, R.W. Parsons, and D.R. Hillman. Association of sleep apnea with myocardial infarction in men. *Lancet* 1990; 336:261–264.

7. Watson, Robert, Glen Greenberg, and Dennis Deptula. Neurophysiological deficits in sleep apnea (abstract). In *Sleep Research,* Vol. 14, p. 136. Edited by Michael Chase. Los Angeles: UCLA Brain Information Service/Brain Research Institute, 1985.

8. Fairbanks, David. Snoring: an overview. In *Snoring and Obstructive Sleep Apnea.* Edited by David Fairbanks, Shiro Fujita, T. Ikematsu, and F.B. Simmons. New York: Raven, 1987.

9. Shepard, John W. Pathophysiology and medical therapy of sleep apnea. *Ear Nose Throat J* 1984 May; 63(5):198–212.

10. Strohl, Kingman P., Colin E. Sullivan, and Nicholas A. Saunders. Sleep apnea syndromes. In *Sleep and Breathing.* Edited by Nicholas A. Saunders and Colin E. Sullivan. Lung Biology in Health and Disease Series, Vol. 21. New York: Marcel Dekker, 1984.

11. Harper, Ronald M. Obstructive sleep apnea. In *Hypoxia, Exercise, and Altitude: Proceedings of the 3rd International Hypoxia Symposium,* pp. 97–105. Progress in Clinical and Biological Research Series, Vol. 136. New York: Liss, 1983.

12. Guilleminault, Christian, and William C. Dement. Sleep apnea syndromes and related sleep disorders. In *Sleep Disorders: Diagnosis and Treatment.* Edited by Robert L. Williams and Ismet Karacan. New York: Wiley, 1978.

13. Kohler U., J. Mayer, J. H. Peter, and P. v. Wichert. Cardiac arrhythmias accompanying sleep apnea activity (SAA) in patients with established sleep apnea and in general outpatients (abstract). In *Sleep Research,* Vol. 14, p. 179. Edited by Michael Chase. Los Angeles: UCLA Brain Information Service/Brain Research Institute, 1985.

14. Jennum, Poul, Kirsten Schultz-Larsen, and Gordon Wildscheidtz. Snoring as a medical risk factor. IV. Relation to lung function and hemoglobin concentration (abstract). In *Sleep Research,* Vol. 14, p. 173. Edited by Michael Chase. Los Angeles: UCLA Brain Information Service/Brain Research Institute, 1985.

15. Podszus, Th., J. Mayer, Th. Penzel, J.H. Peter, P. v. Wichert. Hemodynamics during sleep in patients with sleep apnea (abstract). In *Sleep Research,* Vol. 14, p. 198. Edited by Michael Chase. Los Angeles: UCLA Brain Information Service/Brain Research Institute, 1985.
16. Cartwright, Rosalind, and Sara Knight. Silent partners: the wives of sleep apneic patients. *Sleep* 1987; 10(3):244–248.
17. Guilleminault, Christian, and Elio Lugaresi. *Sleep/Wake Disorders: Natural History, Epidemiology, and Long-Term Evolution.* New York: Raven, 1983.
18. Lavie, Peretz, and A.E. Rubin. Effects of nasal occlusion on respiration in sleep: evidence of inheritability of sleep apnea proneness. *Acta Otolaryngol* (Stockh) 1984 Jan–Feb; 97(1–2):127–130.
19. Young, Terry, Mari Palta, Jerome Dempsey, James Skatrud, Steven Weber, and Safwan Badr. The occurrence of sleep-disordered breathing among middle-aged adults. *N Engl J Med* 1993; 328(17):1230–1235.
20. Dement, William C. *Some Must Watch While Some Must Sleep.* San Francisco: W.H. Freeman, 1972.
21. Orr, William C. Utilization of polysomnography in the assessment of sleep disorders. *Med Clin North Am* 1985; 69(6):1153–1167.
22. Lavie, Peretz. Sleep apnea in industrial workers. In *Sleep/Wake Disorders: Natural History, Epidemiology, and Long-Term Evolution.* New York: Raven, 1983.
23. Hales, Dianne. *The Complete Book of Sleep: How Your Nights Affect Your Days Reading.* North Reading, Mass.: Addison-Wesley, 1981.

*C*hapter 3

1. Dement, William C. *Some Must Watch While Some Must Sleep.* San Francisco: W.H. Freeman, 1972.
2. Randazzo A.C., P.K. Schweitzer, and J.K. Walsh. Cognitive function following 3 nights of sleep restriction in children 10–14. *Sleep* 1998; 21(Suppl):249.
3. Johnson D., D. Thorne, L. Rowland, H. Balkin, et al. The effects of partial sleep deprivation on psychomotor vigilance. *Sleep* 1998; 21(Suppl):204.
4. Shepard, John W. Pathophysiology and medical therapy of sleep apnea. *Ear Nose Throat J* 1984 May; 63(5):198–212.
5. Lugaresi, E., S. Mondini, M. Zucconi, P. Montagna, and F. Cirignotta. Staging of heavy snorers' disease: a proposal. In Proceedings of the 4th International Congress of Sleep Research Satellite Symposium (Bologna). *Bull Eur Physiopathol Respir* 1983; 19(6):590–594.

*C*hapter 4

1. Guilleminault, Christian, M.D. Stanford Sleep Disorders Center, Stanford, California. Interview, 28 March 1986.
2. Jamieson, Andrew, C. Guilleminault, M. Partinen, and M.A. Quera–Salva. Obstructive sleep apnea patients have craniomandibular abnormalities. *Sleep* 1986; 9(4):469–477.
3. Shepard, John W. Pathophysiology and medical therapy of sleep apnea. *Ear Nose Throat J* 1984 May 63(5):198–212.

*C*hapter 5

1. Dement, William. Statement on the Findings and Recommendations of the National Commission on Sleep Disorders Research, Field hearing before U.S. Senate Appropriations Committee, Portland, Oregon, November 4, 1992.

*C*hapter 6

1. Standards of Practice Committee of the American Sleep Disorders Association. Practice parameters for the use of portable recording in the assessment of obstructive sleep apnea. *Sleep* 1994; 17(4):372–377.
2. American Sleep Disorders Association Standards of Practice Committee. Practice parameters for the indications for polysomnography and related procedures. *Sleep* 1997; 20(6):406–422.

*C*hapter 7

1. Colman M.F. Limitations, pitfalls, and risk management in palatopharyngoplasty. In *Snoring and Obstructive Sleep Apnea*. Edited by David Fairbanks, Shiro Fujita, T. Ikematsu, and F.B. Simmons. New York: Raven, 1987.
2. Thawley, Stanley E. Surgical treatment of obstructive sleep apnea. *Med Clin North Am* 1985; 69(6):1337–1357.

3. White, David P., Clifford W. Zwillich, Cheryl K. Pickett, Neil J. Douglas, Larry J. Findley, and John V. Weil. Central sleep apnea: improvement with acetazolamide therapy. *Arch Intern Med* 1982 Oct; 142:1816–1819.

4. Whyte, K.F., G.A. Gould, M.A.A. Airlie, C.M. Shapiro, and N.J. Douglas. Role of protriptyline and acetazolamide in sleep apnea/hypopnea syndrome. *Sleep* 1988; 11(5):463–472.

5. Shore, Eric T., and Richard P. Millman. Central sleep apnea and acetazolamide therapy (letter). *Arch Intern Med* 1983 June; 143:1278, 1280.

6. Guilleminault, Christian, and William C. Dement. Sleep apnea syndromes and related sleep disorders. In *Sleep Disorders: Diagnosis and Treatment.* Edited by Robert L. Williams and Ismet Karacan. New York: Wiley, 1978.

7. Guilleminault, Christian, Johanna van den Hoed, and Merrill M. Mitler. Clinical overview of the sleep apnea syndromes. In *Sleep Apnea Syndromes,* Kroc Foundation Series, Vol. 11. Edited by Christian Guilleminault and William C. Dement. New York: Liss, 1978.

8. Gotfried, Mark H., and Stuart F. Quan. Obstructive sleep apnea—pathogenesis and treatment. *Lung* 1984;162:1–13.

9. Schmidt, H. L-Tryptophan in the treatment of impaired respiration in sleep. In Proceedings of the 4th International Congress of Sleep Research Satellite Symposium (Bologna). *Bull Eur Physiopathol Respir* 1983; 19(6):625–629.

10. Krieger, J., P. Mangin, and D. Kurtz. Effects of almitrine in the treatment of sleep apnea syndromes. In Proceedings of the 4th International Congress of Sleep Research Satellite Symposium (Bologna). *Bull Eur Physiopathol Respir* 1983; 19(6):630.

11. Douglas, N.J., J.J. Connaughton, A.D. Morgan, C.N. Shapiro, N. Pauly, and D.C. Flenly. Effect of almitrine on nocturnal hypoxaemia in chronic bronchitis and emphysema, and in patients with central sleep apnea. In Proceedings of the 4th International Congress of Sleep Research Satellite Symposium (Bologna). *Bull Eur Physiopathol Respir* 1983; 19(6):631.

12. Krieger, J., P. Mangin, and D. Kurtz. Almitrine and sleep apnea. *Lancet* 1982 July 24; 9(8291):210.

13. White, David P. Central sleep apnea. *Med Clin North Am* 1985; 69(6):1205–1219.

14. Meisner H., J.G. Schober, E. Struck, B. Lipowski, P. Mayser, and F. Sebening. Phrenic nerve pacing for the treatment of central hypoventilation syndrome—state of the art and case report. *Thorac Cardiovasc Surgeon* 1983; 31:21–25.

15. Brouillette, Robert T., Michel N. Ilbawi, and Carl E. Hunt. Phrenic nerve pacing in infants and children: a review of experience and report on the usefulness of phrenic nerve stimulation studies. *J Pediatrics* 1983 Jan; 102(1):32–39.

16. Glenn, William W.L., Mildred Phelps, and Larry M. Gersten. Diaphragm pacing in the management of central alveolar hypoventilation. In *Sleep Apnea Syndromes,*

Kroc Foundation Series, Vol. 11. Edited by Christian Guilleminault and William C. Dement. New York: Liss, 1978.

17. Sullivan, Colin E., Michael Berthon–Jones, Faiq G. Issa, and Lorraine Eves. Reversal of obstructive sleep apnoea by continuous positive airway pressure applied through the nares. *Lancet* 1981 April 18; 1(8225):862–865.

18. Issa, Faiq G., and Colin E. Sullivan. Reversal of central apnea using nasal CPAP. *Chest* 1986; 90(2):165–176.

19. Burwell, C. Sidney, Eugene D. Robin, Robert D. Whaley, and Albert G. Bikelman. Extreme obesity associated with alveolar hypoventilation—a Pickwickian syndrome. *Am J Med* 1956; 21:811–818.

20. Jung, Richard, and Wolfgang Kuhlo. Neurophysiological studies of abnormal night sleep in the Pickwickian syndrome. *Progress in Brain Research: Sleep Mechanisms* 1965; 18:140–159.

21. Rinke, Carlotta. Shedding a little light on sleep disorders. *JAMA* 1981 Feb; 245(6):549.

22. Sanders, Mark H., Cynthia A. Gruendl, and Robert M. Rogers. Patient compliance with nasal CPAP therapy for sleep apnea. *Chest* 1986; 90(3):330–333.

23. Cartwright, R.D., and C.F. Samelson. Effects of a non-surgical treatment for obstructive sleep apnea—the tongue-retaining device. *JAMA* 1982; 248(6): 705–709.

24. Cartwright, Rosalind D. Predicting response to the tongue retaining device for sleep apnea syndrome. *Arch Otolaryngol* 1985; 111:385–388.

25. Soll, Bruce A., and Peter T. George. Treatment of obstructive sleep apnea with a nocturnal airway-patency appliance. *N Engl J Med* 1985; 313(6):386, 387.

26. Andrews, J.N., Christian Guilleminault, and R.A. Holdaway. Retaining devices and mandibular positioning appliances. In Proceedings of the 4th International Congress of Sleep Research Satellite Symposium (Bologna). *Bull Eur Physiopathol Respir* 1983; 19(6):611.

27. Avidan, A.Y., Joseph A. Golish, Dudley S. Dinner, et al. The mandibular advancement device for the treatment of obstructive sleep apnea. Abstract C100.K1. *Sleep* 1999; 22(Suppl 1).

28. Parker, Jonathan A., Salim Kathwalla, Susan Ravenscraft, et al. A prospective study evaluating the effectiveness of a mandibular repositioning appliance (PM Positioner) for the treatment of moderate obstructive sleep apnea. Abstract C376.K1. *Sleep* 1999; 22(Suppl 1).

29. Barbosa, Ricardo C., Flavio S. Aloe, Stella M. Taveres, and Ademir B. Silva. Oral appliance treatment: PSG results in 16 mild to severe OSAS subjects. Abstract C502.J. *Sleep* 1999; 22(Suppl 1).

30. American Sleep Disorders Association. Standards of Practice Committee. Practice parameters for the treatment of snoring and obstructive sleep apnea with oral

appliances. *Sleep* 1995; 18(6):511–513.

31. Brownell, L.G., R. Perez-Padilla, P. West, and M.H. Kryger. The role of protriptyline in obstructive sleep apnea. In Proceedings of the 4th International Congress of Sleep Research Satellite Symposium (Bologna). *Bull Eur Physiopathol Respir* 1983; 19(6):621–624.

32. Guilleminault, C., and S. Mondini. Need for multi-diagnostic approaches before considering treatment in obstructive sleep apnea. In Proceedings of the 4th International Congress of Sleep Research Satellite Symposium (Bologna). *Bull Eur Physiopathol Respir* 1983; 19(6):583–589.

33. Smith, Philip L., Edward F. Haponik, Richard P. Allen, and Eugene R. Bleecker. The effects of protriptyline in sleep-disordered breathing. *Am Rev Respir Dis* 1983; 127:8–13.

34. Conway, W., S. Fujita, F. Zorick, K. Sicklesteel, T. Roehrs, R. Wittig, and T. Roth. Uvulopalatopharyngoplasty: one-year follow-up. *Chest* 1985 Sept; 88(3):385–387.

35. Guilleminault, C., B. Hayes, L. Smith, and F.B. Simmons. Palatopharyngoplasty and obstructive sleep apnea syndrome. In Proceedings of the 4th International Congress of Sleep Research Satellite Symposium (Bologna). *Bull Eur Physiopathol Respir* 1983; 19(6):595–599.

36. Katsantonis, George P., James K. Walsh, Paula K. Schweitzer, and William H. Friedman. Further evaluation of uvulopalatopharyngoplasty in the treatment of obstructive sleep apnea syndrome. *Otolaryngol Head Neck Surg* 1985 April; 93(2): 244–250.

37. Fujita, Shiro, William A. Conway, Frank J. Zorick, Jeanne M. Sicklesteel, Timothy A. Roehrs, Robert M. Wittig, and Thomas Roth. Evaluation of the effectiveness of uvulopalatopharyngoplasty. *Laryngoscope* 1985 Jan; 95:70–74.

38. Riley, R., C. Guilleminault, N. Powell, and F. Blair Simmons. Palatopharyngoplasty failure, cephalometric roentgenograms, and obstructive sleep apnea. *Otolaryngol Head Neck Surg* 1985 April; 93(2):240–243.

39. Riley, Robert, Christian Guilleminault, Juan Herran, and Nelson Powell. Cephalometric analyses and flow-volume loops in obstructive sleep apnea patients. *Sleep* 1983; 6(4):303–311.

40. Jamieson, Andrew, C. Guilleminault, M. Partinen, and M.A. Quera–Salva. Obstructive sleep apnea patients have craniomandibular abnormalities. *Sleep* 1986; 9(4):469–477.

41. Moran, W.B. Jr. Obstructive sleep apnea: diagnosis by history, physical exam, and special studies. In *Snoring and Obstructive Sleep Apnea*. Edited by David Fairbanks, Shiro Fujita, T. Ikematsu, and F.B. Simmons. New York: Raven, 1987.

42. Shepard, John W. Jr., Warren B. Gefter, Christian Guilleminault, Eric A. Hoffman, Victor Hoffstein, David W. Hudgel, Paul M. Suratt, and David P. White. Evaluation of the upper airway in patients with obstructive sleep apnea. *Sleep*

1991; 14(4):361–371.

43. Penek, J. Laser-assisted uvulopalatoplasty: the cart before the horse. *Chest* 1995; 107(1):1–3.

44. American Sleep Disorders Association. Standards of Practice Committee. Practice parameters for the use of laser-assisted uvulopalatoplasty. *Sleep* 1994; 17(8):744–748.

45. Wareing M.J., V.P. Callanan, and D.B. Mitchell. Laser assisted uvulopalatoplasty: six and eighteen month results. *J Laryngol Otol* 1998; 112(7):639–641.

46. Powell N.B., R.W. Riley, R.J. Troell, K. Ki, M.B. Blumen, and C. Guilleminault. Radiofrequency volumetric tissue reduction of the palate in subjects with sleep-disordered breathing. *Chest* 1998; 113(5):1163–1174.

47. Powell, Nelson B., and Robert W. Riley. Radiofrequency tongue base reduction in sleep disordered breathing: a pilot study. *Otolaryngol Head Neck Surg* 1998; 119(2):5.

48. Fujita, Shiro, T. Woodson, J.L. Clark, and R. Wittig. Laser midline glossectomy as a treatment for obstructive sleep apnea. *Laryngoscope* 1991; 101:805–809.

49. Mickelson, Samuel A., and Leon Rosenthal. Midline glossectomy and epiglottidectomy for obstructive sleep apnea syndrome. *Laryngoscope* 1997; 107:614-619.

50. Riley, R.W., N.B. Powell, and C. Guilleminault. Obstructive sleep apnea syndrome: a surgical protocol for dynamic upper airway reconstruction. *J Oral Maxillofac Surg* 1993; 51(7):742-747.

51. Riley, R., C. Guilleminault, N. Powell, and S. Derman. Mandibular osteotomy and hyoid bone advancement for obstructive sleep apnea: a case report. *Sleep* 1984; 7(1):79–82

52. Powell, N., C. Guilleminault, R. Riley, and L. Smith. Mandibular advancement and obstructive sleep apnea syndrome. In Proceedings of the 4th International Congress of Sleep Research Satellite Symposium (Bologna). *Bull Eur Physiopathol Respir* 1983; 19(6):607–610.

53. Guilleminault, Christian, F. Blair Simmons, Jorge Motta, Joseph Cummiskey, Mark Rosekind, John S. Schroeder, and William C. Dement. Obstructive sleep apnea syndrome and tracheostomy: long-term follow-up experience. *Arch Intern Med* 1981; 141:985–988.

54. Dye, John P., and L. Jack Faling. Living with a tracheostomy for sleep apnea (letters). *N Engl J Med* 1983 May; 308(19):1167, 1168.

55. Lubin, M.F., H.K. Walker, and R.B. Smith III, eds. *Medical Management of the Surgical Patient.* 2nd ed. London: Butterworths, 1988.

56. Charuzi, Ilan, Amnon Ovnat, Jochanan Peiser, Hedy Saltz, Simon Weitzman, and Peretz Lavie. The effect of surgical weight reduction on sleep quality in obesity-related sleep apnea syndrome. *Surgery* 1985 May; 97(5):535–538.

*C*hapter 8

1. Waldhorn, R.E. Cardiopulmonary consequences of obstructive sleep apnea. In *Snoring and Obstructive Sleep Apnea*. Edited by David Fairbanks, Shiro Fujita, T. Ikematsu, and F.B. Simmons. New York: Raven, 1987.
2. Kryger, Meir H. Sleep apnea: from the needles of Dionysius to continuous positive airway pressure. *Arch Intern Med* 1983 Dec; 143(12):2301–2303.
3. Lavie, Peretz. Nothing new under the moon: historical accounts of sleep apnea syndrome. *Arch Intern Med* 1984 Oct; 144(10):2025–2028.
4. Gastaut, H., C.A. Tassinari, and B. Duron. Polygraphic study of the episodic diurnal and nocturnal (hypnic and respiratory) manifestations of the Pickwick syndrome. *Brain Res* 1966; 2:167–186.
5. Jung, Richard, and Wolfgang Kuhlo. Neurophysiological studies of abnormal night sleep in the Pickwickian syndrome. *Progress in Brain Research: Sleep Mechanisms* 1965; 18:140–159.
6. Charuzi, Ilan, Amnon Ovnat, Jochanan Peiser, Hedy Saltz, Simon Weitzman, and Peretz Lavie. The effect of surgical weight reduction on sleep quality in obesity-related sleep apnea syndrome. *Surgery* 1985 May; 97(5):535–538.
7. Burwell, C. Sidney, Eugene D. Robin, Robert D. Whaley, and Albert G. Bikelman. Extreme obesity associated with alveolar hypoventilation—a Pickwickian syndrome. *Am J Med* 1956; 21:811–818.
8. Sullivan, Colin E., M. Berthon-Jones, and F.G. Issa. Remission of severe obesity-hypoventilation syndrome after short-term treatment during sleep with nasal continuous positive airway pressure. *Am Rev Respir Dis* 1983 July; 128(1):177–181.

*C*hapter 9

1. Limerick, The Countess of. Greetings. In *Sudden Infant Death Syndrome: Proceedings of the 1982 International Research Conference* (Baltimore). Edited by J. Tyson Tildon, Lois M. Roeder, and Alfred Steinschneider. New York: Academic, 1983.
2. Sullivan, Colin E. Personal Communication. 1993. His belief in the link between SIDS and OSA is based on his own recent experience and data from Kahn's group in Belgium.
3. Guilleminault, Christian, and Anstella Robinson. Developmental aspects of sleep and breathing. *Curr Opin Pulm Med* 1996 Nov; 2(6):492-9. Review.

4. McNamara F., and C.E. Sullivan. Evolution of sleep-disordered breathing and sleep in infants. *J Paediatr Child Health* 1998 Feb; 34(1):37-43.

5. Hodgman, Joan E., and Toke Hoppenbrouwers. Cardiorespiratory behavior in infants at increased epidemiological risk for SIDS. In *Sudden Infant Death Syndrome: Proceedings of the 1982 International Research Conference* (Baltimore). Edited by J. Tyson Tildon, Lois M. Roeder, and Alfred Steinschneider. New York: Academic, 1983.

6. Albani, M., K.H.P. Bentele, C. Budde, and F.J. Schulte. Infant sleep apnea profile: preterm vs. term infants. *Eur J Pediatrics* 1985 March; 143(4):261–268.

7. Orsini, A.J., et al. The incidence of post discharge apnea in infants born < 34 weeks gestation with normal inpatient pneumocardiograms. *Pediatr Pulmonol* 1998; 26:443.

8. Pohl, C.A., et al. Role of a screening documented event monitor (DEM) for pathologic apnea and bradycardia in healthy preterm infants. *Pediatr Pulmonol* 1998; 26:445.

9. Stoddard, R.A., and P. Auxier. Predischarge evaluation for apnea and bradycardia in premature infants. *Pediatr Pulmonol* 1998; 26:448

10. Guilleminault, Christian. Sleep apnea in the full-term infant. In *Sleep and Its Disorders in Children*. Edited by Christian Guilleminault. New York: Raven, 1987.

11. National Institutes of Health Consensus Development Conference on Infantile Apnea and Home Monitoring. *Pediatrics* 1987; 79:292-299.

12. Kohlendorfer, Ursula, Stefan Kiechl, and Wolfgang Sperl. Sudden infant death syndrome: risk factor profiles for distinct subgroups. *Am J Epidemiol* 1998; 147(10):960–968.

13. American Academy of Pediatrics. AAP Task Force on Infant Positioning and SIDS. *Pediatrics* 1992; 89(6 Pt 1):1120–1126.

14. Downey, Ralph III, Ronald M. Perkin, and Joanne MacQuarrie. Nasal CPAP use in children with obstructive sleep apnea under 2 years of age. *Pediatr Pulmonol* 1998; 26:443.

15. Golding, Jean, Sylvia Limerick, and Aidan Macfarlane. *Sudden Infant Death: Patterns, Puzzles, and Problems*. Seattle: University of Washington Press, 1985.

*C*hapter 10

1. Ferber, Richard, M.D. *Solve Your Child's Sleep Problems*. New York: Simon & Schuster, 1985.

2. Guilleminault, C., R. Korobkin, and R. Winkle. A review of 50 children with obstructive sleep apnea syndrome. *Lung* 1981; 159:275–287.

3. Wilkinson, A.R., M.S. McCormick, A.P. Freeland, and D. Pickering. Electrocardiographic signs of pulmonary hypertension in children who snore. *Br Med J* 1981; 282:1579–1582.

4. Guilleminault, Christian. Obstructive sleep apnea syndrome in children. In *Sleep and Its Disorders in Children*. Edited by Christian Guilleminault. New York: Raven, 1987.

5. Guilleminault, Christian, and Ronald Ariagno. Apnea during sleep in infants and children. In *Principles and Practice of Sleep Medicine*. Edited by Meir H. Kryger, Thomas Roth, and William C. Dement. Philadelphia: W.B. Saunders, 1989.

*C*hapter 11

1. Prinz, Patricia N., and Murray Raskind. Aging and sleep disorders. In *Sleep Disorders: Diagnosis and Treatment*. Edited by Robert L. Williams and Ismet Karacan. New York: Wiley, 1978.

2. Ancoli-Israel, Sonia, Daniel F. Kripke, William Mason, and Oscar J. Kaplan. Sleep apnea and periodic movements in an aging sample. *J Gerontol* 1985; 40(4): 419–425.

3. Carskadon, Mary A., and William C. Dement. Respiration during sleep in the aged human. *J Gerontol* 1981; 36(4):420–423.

4. Bliwise, Donald L., and Ralph A. Pascualy. Sleep-related respiratory disturbance in elderly persons. *Compr Ther* 1984; 10(7):8–14.

*C*hapter 14

1. Edinger, J.D., and Radtke, R.A. Use of In vivo desensitization to treat a patient's claustrophobic response to nasal CPAP. *Sleep* 1993; 16(7):678–680.

*C*hapter 15

1. Norman, Susan E., and Martin A. Cohn. Follow-up care at sleep disorders centers: a commitment beyond diagnosis (letter). *Sleep* 1985; 8(1):71–73.

Chapter 16

1. Sullivan, Colin E., Michael Berthon-Jones, Faiq G. Issa, and Lorraine Eves. Reversal of obstructive sleep apnoea by continuous positive airway pressure applied through the nares. *Lancet* 1981 April 18; 1(8225):862–865.
2. Dexter, D. Jr. Magnetic therapy is ineffective for the treatment of snoring and obstructive sleep apnea syndrome. *Wis Med J* 1997 Mar; 96(3):35–37.

Glossary

adenoids Similar to tonsils, but located behind and above the tonsils

airway The passage through which air travels as it moves to and from your lungs; your airway includes nose and mouth, throat, and the bronchial tubes that lead to your lungs

angina pectoris Chest pain that occurs when the heart muscle does not get enough oxygen

apnea Failure to move air in and out of your airway

apnea event Failure to breathe that lasts for more than 10 seconds

apnea index The number of apnea events per hour; a measure of the severity of sleep apnea

apnea-plus-hypopnea index The total number of apnea and hypopnea events per hour; a measure of the severity of sleep apnea

arrhythmia Variation from the normal rhythm of the heartbeat

breathing center The center in your brain that controls the speed and forcefulness of your breathing

CPAP Continuous positive airway pressure; a breathing system used to treat obstructive sleep apnea and other respiratory disorders

carbon dioxide The waste gas produced by your body; it is removed from your blood stream in the lungs and leaves the body when you exhale

cardiovascular Pertaining to the heart or circulatory system

carotid body A sensory structure in the carotid artery in the neck that measures the amount of oxygen in your blood and sends signals to the breathing center in your brain

central sleep apnea Sleep apnea that is caused by some irregularity in the brain's control of breathing

cephalometry Measurement of the size and location of the structures in the head using X-rays or other imaging systems

cuirass A breathing device that fits over a patient's chest and helps him breathe; sometimes used to treat central sleep apnea

deviated septum An irregularly shaped nasal septum; may partly block the passage of air and interfere with breathing; see nasal septum

diaphragm The muscular wall that separates the chest cavity from the abdominal cavity; your diaphragm is part of your breathing system; the downward contraction of the diaphragm muscles allows your lungs to expand and fill with air

EDS Excessive daytime sleepiness

ENT specialist Ear, nose, and throat specialist; also called an otolaryngologist

gastric bypass A surgical procedure in which the stomach is stapled to make it smaller; used to promote weight loss in morbidly obese patients

hypertension High blood pressure

hypopnea Shallow breathing in which the airflow in and out of the airway is less than half of normal

larynx The "voice box"; the structure in the lower throat that contains the vocal cords; the Adam's apple is the front of your larynx

LAUP Laser assisted uvulopalatoplasty; laser surgery performed on the soft palate to reduce snoring; not recommended for sleep apnea

mandible Lower jawbone

mandibular reconstruction Surgery to reshape the lower jaw

maxilla Upper jawbone

maxillofacial surgery Surgery on the upper jaw and face

medulla, or medulla oblongata A deep, primitive part of the brain; sensors that detect carbon dioxide are located here; these sensors are involved in your breathing reflex

mixed sleep apnea Sleep apnea that is a combination of obstructive and central apnea

nREM sleep Non-REM sleep; see REM sleep

nasal septum The divider between the right and the left nose cavities; it is made up of bone, cartilage, and soft tissue

neurologic Pertaining to the nervous system

nocturnal Occurring at night

obese Having a weight of more than 20% above the ideal body weight

obstructive sleep apnea Sleep apnea caused by a blockage of the airway

OPAP™ Oral pressure appliance; a small mouthpiece that can be worn either by itself or connected to CPAP tubing and a CPAP machine

otolaryngologist An ear, nose, and throat specialist; also called an ENT specialist

oxygen A gas that makes up 20% of the air your breathe; it is picked up in your lungs by red blood cells and carried throughout your body; all your body's cells need oxygen in order to live

oxygen saturation The amount of oxygen being carried in your blood; often used as a measure of the severity of sleep apnea; normal oxygen saturation is about 95%, with some decrease with age

pharynx The part of the throat just behind the mouth

polycythemia An abnormal excess of red blood cells

polysomnography The recording of a person's breathing, heartbeat, brain activity, body movements, and other physiologic signs during sleep

pulmonary Pertaining to the lungs

RDI Respiratory Disturbance Index; a measure of the severity of sleep apnea; equal to the number of apneas plus hypopneas, divided by total sleep time, and multiplied by 60

red blood cells The cells that carry oxygen through the bloodstream

REM sleep The "rapid eye movement" stage of sleep; the "active" stage of sleep during which the most vivid dreams occur

set point The amount of carbon dioxide or oxygen in your blood that triggers the breathing center to make you inhale

sleep apnea A condition in which a person stops breathing while asleep

sleep latency The amount of time it takes for you to fall asleep; indicates the degree of excessive daytime sleepiness

soft palate The flexible back part of the roof of your mouth

Somnoplasty™ A surgical technique for reducing snoring by using radio frequency energy

tonsils A pair of small glands located at the back of the mouth, on either side of the opening into the throat

UARS See upper airway resistance syndrome

UPPP Uvulopalatopharyngoplasty; a type of surgery sometimes used to treat snoring and obstructive sleep apnea.

upper airway resistance syndrome A type of sleep-disordered breathing associated with arousals from sleep; sometimes called respiratory effort–related arousals (RERAs)

uvula The dangly, tongue-shaped tab that hangs down from the soft palate at the back of your mouth

Index

Note: boldface numbers indicate illustrations

Breathing/lung problems, 40, 50
Broadbent, W.H., earliest description of sleep apnea, 20

Caffeine, 163
Capitated insurance plans, 165
Carbon dioxide/oxygen levels during sleep, 31, 39
Carotid bodies as nerve sensors for oxygen, 30–31
Cataplexy, 22
Causes of sleep apnea, 37–45
Central apnea, 38, 39–40, **41**
  childhood/adolescent sleep apnea, 150
Changing sleep position, 91
Childhood/adolescent sleep apnea, 149–156, 149
  attention-deficit hyperactivity disorder (ADHD) and, 151
  behavior problems as a symptom of, 150
  causes of, 150
  central apnea in, 150
  complications of, 151
  computerized tomography (CAT) scan test for, 153
  CPAP treatment for, 154
  diagnosis of, 152–154
  mixed apnea in, 150
  multiple sleep latency test (MSLT) for, 153
  obesity in, 150, 151, 155
  obstructive apnea in, 150
  school performance as a symptom of, 150
  symptoms of, 150–152
  testing for, 152–154
  tonsils and, 149–150
  treatments for, 154–155
  uvulopalatopharyngoplasty (UPPP) in, 155
  weight loss treatment for, 155
Circulation problems, 16
Claustrophobia and mask removal during CPAP, 193
Clomipramine, 86
Complications of sleep apnea, 2, 20, 50
Computerized tomography (CAT) scan test, 153
Concentration problems, 18, 27
Confusion, 18
Congestive heart failure, 20

childhood/adolescent sleep apnea and, 150
  treatment for, 90–91
Morison, A., 19th century physician, 134
Multiple Sleep Latency Test (MSLT), 53, 68–69, 76
  childhood/adolescent sleep apnea, 153
Muscular dystrophy, 39

Naloxone, 87
Napping, 163
Narcolepsy, 21, 22, 48
Nasal bi-pressure therapy (BiPAP™) in, 90
Nasal congestion, 19, 34, 42
  from CPAP, 194
Nasal surgery, 110
Nellcor Puritan Bennett, CPAP manufacturer, 179–180, 191
Nocturnal myoclonus (restless legs syndrome), 21, 22, 161
Non-REM (NREM) sleep in normal sleep, 28–29
Nonsurgical options in treating sleep apnea, 81
Normal sleep, 25–35
  amount of sleep required, 26, 28
  breathing centers of brain in, 30
  breathing during, 30–35
  breathing muscle action during, 32
  breathing patterns during, **33**
  breathing reflexes in, 30
  carbon dioxide/oxygen levels during, 31
  carotid bodies as nerve sensors for oxygen in, 30–31
  changes in sleep patterns with age, **27**, 157–159, **158**
  development of sleep-disordered breathing from, 34–35
  elderly sleep patterns, **27**, 157–159, **158**
  medulla as oxygen sensor during, 31
  myths about sleep and aging, 160
  non-REM (NREM) sleep in, 28–29
  oxygen "set points" in, 30–32
  physical changes during sleep, 28–29
  physiologic benefits of normal sleep, 26
  quality of sleep in, 28
  rapid eye movement (REM) sleep in, 28–29
  "shift work" and, 26
  "sleep debt" and, 28